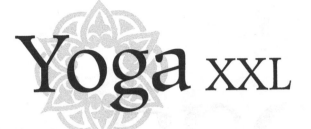

Yoga XXL

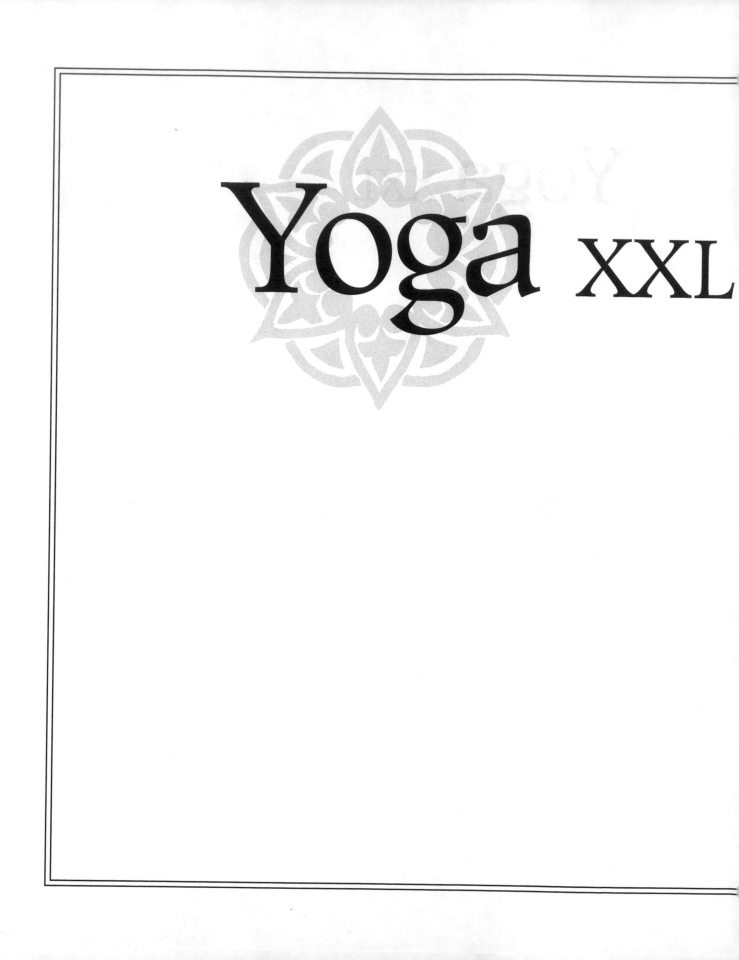

Yoga XXL

A Journey to Health
for Bigger People

INGRID KOLLAK, RN, PhD

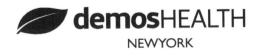
demosHEALTH
NEWYORK

Visit our website at www.demoshealth.com

ISBN: 978-1-936303-48-9
e-book ISBN: 978-1-61705-168-5

Acquisitions Editor: Julia Pastore
Compositor: diacriTech

Medical information provided by Demos Health, in the absence of a visit with a health care professional, must be considered as an educational service only. This book is not designed to replace a physician's independent judgment about the appropriateness or risks of a procedure or therapy for a given patient. Our purpose is to provide you with information that will help you make your own health care decisions.

The information and opinions provided here are believed to be accurate and sound, based on the best judgment available to the authors, editors, and publisher, but readers who fail to consult appropriate health authorities assume the risk of injuries. The publisher is not responsible for errors or omissions. The editors and publisher welcome any reader to report to the publisher any discrepancies or inaccuracies noticed.

Library of Congress Cataloging-in-Publication Data
Kollak, Ingrid.
  Yoga XXL : a journey to health for bigger people / Ingrid Kollak, RN, PhD.
    pages cm
  Includes bibliographical references and index.
  ISBN 978-1-936303-48-9
  1. Weight loss. 2. Yoga. 3. Reducing exercises. I. Title. II. Title:
Yoga seventy. III. Title: Yoga 70.
  RM222.2.K5765 2013
  613.7'046—dc23

                              2013014560

Special discounts on bulk quantities of Demos Health books are available to corporations, professional associations, pharmaceutical companies, health care organizations, and other qualifying groups. For details, please contact:

Special Sales Department
Demos Medical Publishing, LLC
11 West 42nd Street, 15th Floor
New York, NY 10036
Phone: 800-532-8663 or 212-683-0072
Fax: 212-941-7842
E-mail: specialsales@demosmedpub.com

Printed in the United States of America by Bang Printing.
13 14 15 16 17 / 5 4 3 2 1

Also by Ingrid Kollak, RN, PhD

Yoga for Nurses

Yoga and Breast Cancer

The only people who stay truly alive are those who take more pleasure in knowledge, including self-knowledge, than in external acclaim.

—Margarete Mitscherlich

Contents

PART I

HOW TO USE THIS BOOK

PART II

YOGA FOR PEOPLE WITH BIGGER BODIES

CHAPTER 9. STANDING POSTURES AND BOWS   107

CHAPTER 10. STANDING POSTURES WITH ROTATIONS   123

CHAPTER 11. BALANCING POSTURES   133

CHAPTER 12. INVERSIONS   141

PART III

POSTURES IN FLOWING MOTION

PART IV

ROUTINES TO HELP YOU DEVELOP A DAILY YOGA PRACTICE

Foreword

Some readers of this book will likely skip past the introductory text (including this foreword!) and head straight for the photos and exercises that will get them moving and stretching. I say, good for them. Those like me, however, will want to revel first in the encouraging, informative, and body-positive chapter at the front of the book. And I'll confess to especially liking the pictures: I loved seeing photos of real XXL yogis captioned with their confident assertions that size is no barrier to enjoying great health and satisfying physical activity.

While these notions may startle some, they seem obvious to me. You see, I have built an entire career—as a nutrition professor, therapist, exercise physiologist, researcher and author—on the premises of Health at Every Size, or HAES®. HAES precepts rest on voluminous evidence that we are healthiest when we appreciate and care for the bodies we're in and most likely to achieve good health when we abandon a focus on weight-loss. We can achieve fitness, good nutrition, and well-being, it turns out, regardless of our shape or dimensions.

HAES recognizes that there can no more be a single "normal" or healthy body shape or weight than there could be a perfect, healthy height or ear shape. Body Mass Index is not destiny, nor is it a sound measure of health. (U.S. government data from the Centers for Disease Control mirrors that of many other studies, showing, in fact, that a little "extra" body weight is associated with *increased* longevity.)

Now, it's easier to act on all this if we recognize, and learn to reject, our society's prevailing fat stigma. We might readily enough accept that a fat body (in the HAES community, we use that word proudly:

nothing wrong with fat) can be a healthy body, but find it harder to get used to the idea that it can also be a beautiful one. Yet, we can learn to admire bodies in a variety of shapes, including our own—adorning them and taking pride in their curves as well as for all that they do for us. Without such acceptance, it's hard to let go of diet culture and embrace the imperative of self-care.

One basic element of that care is learning to feed ourselves well, and the other is embracing physical activity. Studies show that our culture's emphasis on weight loss tends to be part of the problem rather than any kind of solution. We see increasingly that learning to eat without rules, without trying to "control" our appetites, actually leads to more nutritious eating and greater satisfaction. "Your body is the best nutritionist you'll ever know" is a basic precept of my next book, *Eat Well: For Your Self, for the World*. That's why HAES focuses on eating "intuitively," learning to let internal signals take charge—or relearning, actually, since we did it as babies.

As for the joy and benefits of finding movement you like, physical activity is available to all people and worthwhile in its own right, even if it never causes anyone to "drop" an ounce. Whether it's dance you like, bowling, walking, swimming, games, aerobics, hula hoops, or of course, *yoga*, anyone can enjoy the good feelings that can come from putting our bodies to work. Books like this one do so much to open doors—and yoga studios, running clubs, gyms and hearts—to this uplifting idea.

Ingrid starts with the HAES-friendly premise that exercising for well-being is better, and more effective, than exercising for slimming purposes. She explains how yoga practice can meet the all-important HAES priority of caring well for the body you're in, and stresses that thinness conveys no special access to fitness and health. "Despite what you might see in the media," she explains, "yoga is not the exclusive territory of the lean and limber." (I find it puzzling, in fact, that some of the same folks who enthuse about and encourage yoga's accessibility to people of all ages, from small children to the elderly, overlook or even actively exclude larger people.)

Yoga XXL inspires through these liberating ideas and its profiles of happily practicing large-sized yogis. The advice, photos, and instructions are clear and easy to follow. And for those with physical barriers to certain exercises or moves, it includes techniques like props and modifications to make the exercises safe and possible. The advice found here will help just about anyone, large or small, old or young, experienced or out of shape, seeking fitness and a measure of serenity through yoga practice.

As Ingrid makes clear, you don't have to be thin (or young, or hip, or dressed in fancy gear) to enjoy and grow through yoga. And you also don't have to be XXL to enjoy and get the most out of this book.

Linda Bacon, PhD
www.LindaBacon.org

Acknowledgments

Yoga does not depend on size, age, or weight. Yoga can be practiced by everyone who enjoys it. This is one of the most common sentiments expressed by the yoga students with bigger bodies whom I interviewed for this book. Their attitudes, as well as their ability to practice all kinds of yoga postures, underline the intention of this book to focus on healthy yogis of all sizes.

I could not have written this book without the help of a group of women who have been practicing yoga together for many years: Anika, Brigitte, Céline, Denise, Doris, and Silke. My special thanks go to Gabi Lutterbeck, teacher of this group of yoga students, who strongly supports a new yoga culture with her class *Yoga for Big People*. I had expert help from photographer Marta Mlejnek to obtain the many different yoga postures included in this book. Special thanks go to Julia Pastore who helped make this an enjoyable book to read.

PART
I

HOW TO USE THIS BOOK

Yoga Is for Everybody

Everyone, no matter her or his size, shape, or physical fitness, can do yoga and experience its health benefits. My own experience with yoga began at the end of the 1990s when my work and private life were radically affected by a slipped disc. I suffered unbelievable pain, couldn't walk, couldn't sit, and couldn't sleep. This was an awful time, but it gave me the chance to ask myself how I wanted my life to continue. I decided it was time to take better care of myself, do more of the work I like, and cooperate more with people who are supportive. A steady yoga practice helped me to become fitter and to achieve my goals. A year later I started to train to become a yoga teacher and continued to be a researcher and professor.

Through professional engagements, I extended my regular practice as a yoga teacher and did yoga twice a week for eighteen months with women who had undergone breast cancer surgery. I watched the remarkable effects yoga had on these women. Physically, they were more flexible—some even more flexible than before their surgery. But the most profound change I witnessed was in their attitude and outlook. Participants who seemed absentminded and unfocused at the start of class looked self-assured, seemed confident, and were eager to make plans for the future at the end of class. This experience confirmed my belief that yoga has a positive impact beyond its direct physical health benefits.

Working on this book with bigger yoga students and models supported my view. Once again I learned that yoga provides the encouraging feeling of power—physically and mentally—and teaches us to appreciate our bodies and to practice successful self-care. Despite what you might see in the media, yoga is not the exclusive territory of the lean and limber. Yoga *is* suitable for everybody.

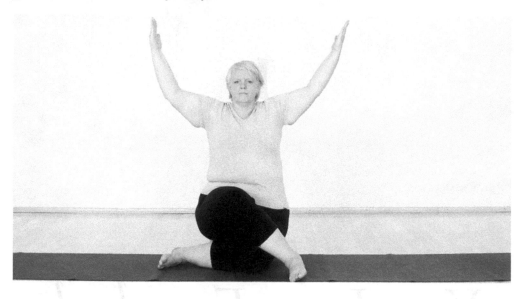

"Yoga does not depend on size, age, or weight. Yoga can be practiced by everyone who enjoys it."
—Silke

HEALTHY YOGIS COME IN ALL SIZES

There is a new zest in yoga these days as more people with bigger bodies show up in yoga classes. They are looking for pleasurable and noncompetitive yoga. And they are in good company with people of all ages and diverse backgrounds who are looking for a healthier approach toward yoga. Enormously effective is the large community of yoga students and teachers who believe in yoga as a supportive culture for people of all sizes, shapes, colors, sexes, and ages. Part of this open culture is the new knowledge of modified postures and useful props.

This yoga book promotes health. Studies have found that the ruling focus on weight loss is ineffective and leads to serious consequences. On an individual level, we experience a preoccupation with food and eating disorders. On a social level, we experience weight stigmatization and a growing industry of dieting products.

It is easier for bigger people to become fit than it is to become slim. Instead of waiting for the next diet plan, you will feel more satisfaction improving your health right now. Yoga students of diverse sizes experience multidimensional well-being and health. Yoga improves both physical and emotional well-being. Backaches, tight muscles, and tension headaches can be remedied through yoga exercises. Yoga also helps to ease stress and recurring troubling thoughts. When practicing yoga, the mind/body connection becomes obvious.

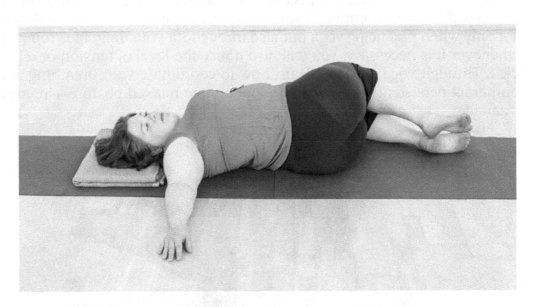

"When I show up at the doctor's office, people are surprised by my normal blood pressure. It is funny how deeply rooted is the belief that health only comes in small bodies."

—Anika

HOW YOGA WORKS

At the beginning of your yoga practice, you will notice the physical benefits. You need strength and attention to do yoga postures in motion or as static exercises and, after a while, you will recognize that you have gained muscle strength, increased flexibility, and achieved better balance. You will feel healthier doing yoga and more in touch with your body. This is particularly liberating in a society that views bigger bodies as unacceptable.

When you are practicing yoga postures, you are concentrating on your body; you become aware of how your breath is leading your movements. Synchronized breathing and moving keep you focused, help you to relax, and shift your thinking from daily chores. You will feel emotionally and physically better grounded. At the end of a class or practice session, your mind will be calmer and clearer. This positive feeling can last for some time and it will boost your energy to accomplish what you must as well as what you love. Yoga provides a feeling of well-being that is far too good to be measured in calories.

BODY AWARENESS

Through the practice of yoga, you will become more aware of your body and your physical well-being. You will become attentive to your posture, and, in this way, you will notice poor postures not only when practicing yoga but also throughout your daily life. You will be able to adjust whenever it is necessary. You will also notice the level of tension or relaxation in your muscles. Through yoga, you will learn how to coordinate your breathing and movement to counteract persistent tensions and adopt a more relaxed posture—in yoga as well as in everyday life.

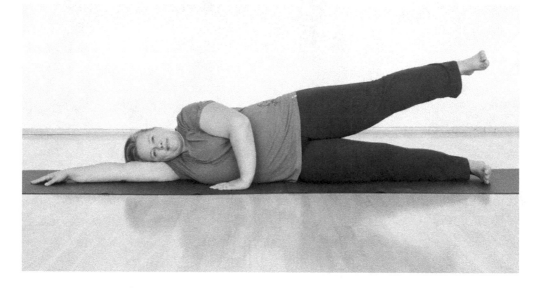

SELF-AWARENESS AND SELF-RELIANCE

In the beginning, you will focus your attention on your body, but as your yoga practice develops, you will learn to recognize your thoughts and feelings while doing yoga postures. In this way, your physical and mental activities will be working in the same direction. This is very important and is one of the main sources of energy and power deriving from yoga. It is vital to recognize these energizing moments. Therefore, this book marks pauses in the midst of or at the end of every yoga exercise. If you are able to understand how you obtained a certain feeling of energy or relaxation, you will be better able to induce those feelings during your everyday life.

Through yoga you will learn to master new skills and build confidence in your abilities and capacity to successfully master all challenges—on the yoga mat and beyond.

2

Getting Started

The yoga exercises described in this book have already been tested on groups of women and men participating in mixed classes and classes for people with bigger bodies. They are distinct variations on classical yoga postures (asana). They can be done in groups or as an individual daily yoga practice at home. They can also be done in between and included in daily routines. It does not matter if you practice alone or in a group with a regular and conscious practice; in any event, you will feel enduring benefits.

GENERAL NOTES OF CAUTION

Before beginning any new exercise practice, speak to your health care provider and determine your personal health status. It is important to know how healthy you really are and whether you have any health issues or undiagnosed health problems. You should pay particular attention to uncontrolled high blood pressure, diabetes, and existing joint or muscle problems.

Pregnant women should only do yoga exercises specifically tailored for their condition. People with glaucoma, a detached retina, ear inflammation, or high blood pressure should keep their heads above heart level. If you feel acute pain, do relaxing postures, and do not fight the pain. After longer breaks (i.e., injury, sickness, and surgical treatment), slowly restart your yoga practice. If you have an abdominal hernia or any injury or inflammation in your back or abdomen, or if you have sciatica, consult your health care practitioner before you start practicing.

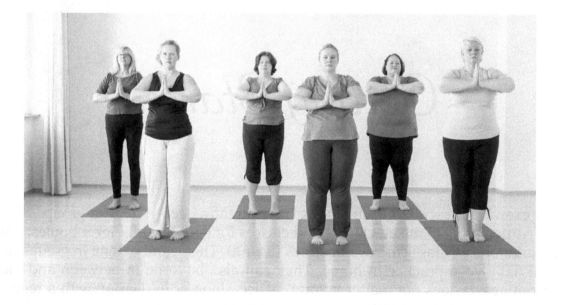

BREATHING AND MOVING

When practicing yoga, breathing should be even, complete, and synchronous with the movement. To maintain a harmony of breathing and moving during long stretches of practicing yoga, it is essential to breathe evenly, in and out, through your nose. This breathing provides the necessary strength to get into the posture, stretch muscles, and hold the posture. The breathing also shows the amount of energy necessary for a posture. You should never be out of breath while practicing yoga. Always practice on a level that allows you to breathe evenly.

There are breathing exercises that make the breath audible and clarify whether breathing and movement are proceeding synchronously. Some yoga schools use humming sounds to let you sense the synchronicity of breathing and moving. The sound should be audible to the very end of the movement. Conscious breathing also helps you to stay focused. Notice how long you can focus on your breath streaming past your nostrils: notice the fresh air streaming into your nose and the warm air streaming out of your nose.

CLOTHING AND EQUIPMENT

Wear comfortable clothes, such as sweatpants and T-shirts, that have a relaxed fit. Practice yoga with bare foot so that you can distribute your weight evenly on your soles, strengthen your foot muscles, feel the outer sides of your feet on the ground, and have a safe posture. At work you can practice yoga in your normal working clothes and shoes as long as they allow stretches and bends.

Use a nonslip yoga mat or exercise on the floor, and use a blanket for all relaxing breathing and concentrating exercises. Roll up a blanket and use it as a bolster for your knees or as a support for your head if you prefer or need it. You do not need to buy specialized props. Books, belts, blankets, and towels can all be used instead, and I have noted these props in the description of each posture.

FINDING THE RIGHT YOGA CLASS

In addition to your individual practice, you may enjoy a class. Surrounded by other people, you can truly feel the power and joy of yoga. There are many different schools and styles of yoga. In the resources section of this book, you will find a list of yoga traditions and their websites to help you to decide which approach is best for you.

Yoga has been changing from a guru-oriented teaching culture to a student-oriented learning one, conducted in a supportive setting. Teachers are more sensitive to the needs of their students, and schools are better equipped to support students with various demands. Appropriate responses to a class should be invigoration, calm, and satisfaction. Inappropriate responses would be stress, agitation, or physical discomfort.

Some people prefer yoga classes specifically for people with large bodies. Others prefer mixed classes. Others attend both types of classes. Choose the class, teacher, and situation that feels best to you and that will make you want to attend regularly.

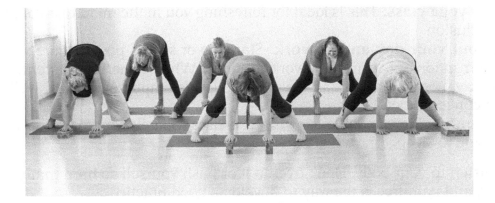

"It is important not to overburden oneself and not to forcefully keep up with others and to enjoy yoga. It was good for me to start with a yoga group for large people."

—Celine

There are minimum standards for the education and qualification of yoga teaching. The professional organization of yoga teachers has a list of trained yoga teachers.

Here are some questions to ask the yoga instructor when considering a yoga class:

- What are your qualifications? How long have you been teaching? Do you have any specialized training?
- How large is the class?
- Do you offer individual support and modifications of classical yoga postures during the class?
- Do you have the knowledge and equipment to fit my needs?
- What is your attitude toward participants with bigger bodies?
- Do you offer a free trial class?

DEVELOP YOUR OWN YOGA PRACTICE

It is vital to develop a conscious yoga practice. Start exercising with your eyes open, closing them only at the end of an exercise or after you worked on the first side, if it helps you to feel the effects. After some practice, you might even prefer to exercise with your eyes closed.

Always start the exercises on the same side of the body.

Practicing yoga regularly is the key to success. It is ideal to practice at the same place and at the same time. This makes it easier to notice your improvements and become aware of your current strengths and weaknesses.

- **In the morning:** If you practice yoga directly after waking up, you will experience the benefits of stretched muscles, flexible joints, increased blood circulation, and improved mood all day.
- **A regular yoga class:** This is ideal for refreshing you in the middle of your workday or at its conclusion.
- **Throughout your day and at work:** Standing or seated postures are well suited for short interruptions of your daily work routines. When done intermittently during the working day, yoga exercises can lower stress levels, improve physical well-being, and increase concentration levels.
- **In the evening:** Slow and relaxing yoga exercises will help you to find peace and quiet before going to sleep.

Always listen to your body. Don't overdo it or push yourself so hard that you feel pain. Slow, steady, and pain-free is the way to develop a good practice.

Each time that you practice a posture, you will better understand its effect on your body and learn to adapt postures to your needs. Experienced yoga students know when they need a special stretch, an extra bend, or a certain resting posture. To become an expert, it is vital that you practice yoga consistently and with awareness. From the beginning, keep to your yoga schedule and your rhythm, and pay attention to what your body is telling you. As you develop your daily practice, consider alternating new or challenging exercises with well-known or easier postures.

Your enjoyment of yoga will increase as your experience grows. You will find that you are able to do more with less exertion and that the regular repetition of postures will become more stimulating. Once you are able to achieve a certain posture, you will be able to concentrate more on the effect it has on your body and mood and less on the physical requirements necessary to maintain it.

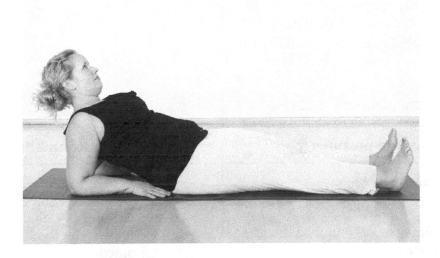

KEEPING A PERSONAL JOURNAL

A personal journal can be of help while you are learning yoga. It gives you a place to write down your goals, determine options for achieving those goals, formulate a plan of action, document your progress, and chronicle your thoughts and feelings.

Divide a notebook or a document file on your computer into two columns: one in which you note what you want to achieve and when and the other in which you write down what you have done, including any comments, thoughts, and ideas. Make sure that your goals are specific; instead of writing "less pain" or "feel better," write "keep my spine stretched" or "reduce neck pain." Your actions should be something that you want to do, that you realistically can do, and that bring you closer to a healthier life.

When coming up with an action plan, ask yourself:

- What do I want to achieve?
- Which postures am I going to practice?
- How often and how much do I want to practice?
- At what time do I want to practice?

When evaluating your actions, recognize new skills, changes in energy, and alterations in your well-being. Don't forget to credit your successes, and use them to bolster further progress. Note:

- How often you practice
- The effects on your body
- Comparisons before and after the exercise
- Differences between the sides of your body
- Improvements to your flexibility
- The effects of any props
- Thoughts you have while practicing
- Progress and obstacles to your daily practice

Examples:

1. Goals, matching postures, and results

Goals and postures	Results
Easing pain in my lower back Knees to chest Twelve movements per session, two times per day during one week • After wake up • During morning break at work	Missed my wake-up exercise on Monday and Tuesday because I stayed in bed too long. Since Wednesday, changed to bedtime exercises. Much easier to do! Back feels better after practicing at work and when lying in bed. Slept well!

2. Goals, postures, and different ways to get results

Goals, postures	Results
Easing pain in the lower back Knees to chest on a mat Twelve movements per session, two times per day during week one: • After wake up • Variation on the chair during morning break	The knees to chest helps a lot to stretch and get started. No back pain on Saturday after a two-hour visit at the museum!
Easing pain in the lower back Folded leaf posture in bed Keep the posture for twelve inhalations and exhalations per session, two times per day during week two: • After wake up • Before falling asleep	The folded leaf posture is comfy but not as effective as the knees to chest. At nighttime the folded leaf posture is a treat. I will keep to it as well as knees to the chest in the morning.

A journal will help you to notice a new competence, stay on track, and use yoga as a way to enhance your well-being. Notice your progress and honor it.

THE STRUCTURE OF THIS BOOK

Each chapter of this book includes detailed entries for several yoga postures. Postures may have two forms: static (without movement) and dynamic (including movement). Each entry includes:

Purposes: This section discusses specific benefits of the posture.

Notes of caution and contraindications: This part covers conditions or factors that may influence your capacity to perform the posture.

Alignments: This section describes the optimal alignment for your body in this posture so that skeletal bones are efficiently used and muscles have to do less work for the same effect. In all basic postures, the spinal column is stretched out from your pelvis to the crown of your head. In supine postures (lying down on your back), your chin points toward your chest. In seated or standing postures, your chin is parallel to the ground. Your shoulders, arms, face, and tongue are all relaxed.

What to do: This part describes step-by-step instructions for positioning your body and the corresponding breathing techniques. As a beginner, complete six deep inhalations and exhalations, the equivalent of six complete movements.

Possible variations: This section details ways to adapt the postures to accommodate all body types.

Photos: In this part, you can visualize the explained yoga postures and exercise on your own at home as well as at work.

You do not need to start at the beginning of this book and continue cover to cover (although you certainly can). Consider a particular tension in your body that you would like to release, and find postures that address it. Turn to Part IV with suggested practices to address some of the most common issues and complaints, including how to boost your energy and counteract stress.

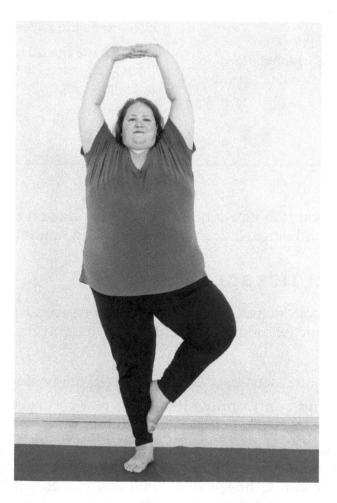

"I want people to look at me and think: If she can do it, I can do it too."
—Doris

YOGA IS JOY

Old yoga texts advise us to do yoga unintentionally—and it is good advice. Start practicing yoga and find out what it does for you. Think of your own experience learning how to write. When you first started writing, you had no clue where your new competence would lead you, but you knew that writing was an important foundation for a lot of things—as yoga is.

The moment you perceive the effects of yoga on the different levels of feeling and understanding I have described, you will enjoy the full measure of its physical and mental pleasures—during practice and beyond. Yoga is bhoga (joy)!

PART
II

YOGA FOR PEOPLE WITH

BIGGER BODIES

3

Postures Lying on the Back (Supine)

Supine postures are those you do lying with your back on the floor and your face up. All of these postures strengthen your muscles and enhance your mobility of joints in a secure basic position. Because you do these postures stretched out on your back, it is easy to keep proper alignment.

These postures help to realign vertebrae and joints and are very effective for people who suffer from back problems as a result of poor posture and weak muscles. Soreness in the upper spine may result in a stiff neck or lack of motion in the head. If the problem is in the lower back, sudden pain and the inability to move may result.

It is important for people with high blood pressure or eye or ear conditions to use a cushion or folded blanket to keep the head above heart level. This chapter includes both static and dynamic exercises.

SUPINE STARTING POSTURE

All supine postures start from this basic position in which your body is stretched out completely, and your arms rest along the sides of your body.

Purposes

The supine starting posture helps you to concentrate and begin your yoga practice. It sharpens your focus on your position, breath, and concentration. As you gain experience, you will find that by taking this position, you immediately become aware of your body alignment, the depth and rhythm of your breathing, and your thoughts, feelings, and mood. When you return to this starting posture between exercises or after the first half of an exercise, you will have the opportunity to assess how your body feels compared to before the exercise.

Notes of Caution and Contraindications

Place your head on a cushion or folded blanket if you suffer from high blood pressure or eye or ear conditions.

Alignments

Your back is fully stretched out on the mat. Your chin is lowered toward your chest to completely stretch your neck.

What to Do

- Lie down on your mat.
- Stretch your neck with your chin pointing toward your chest.
- Stretch your back and your legs.
- Stretch out your arms next to your body with the palms facing downward.
- Let your face, lips, and tongue muscles relax.
- Breathe in and out deeply through your nose.

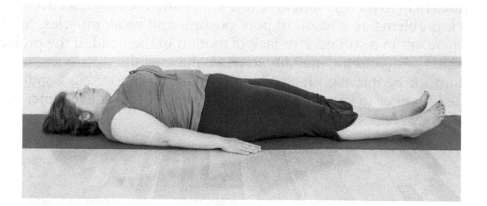

Variation with a Cushion under Your Head

If you have high blood pressure or ear or eye conditions, use a bolster under your head to keep it above your heart level.

■ Place your head on a cushion or folded blanket.

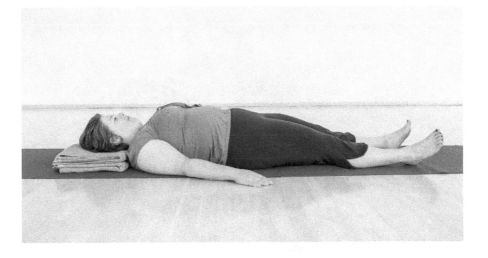

Variation with a Cushion under Your Knees

If you have difficulty stretching your legs or if the lower part of your back is not completely flat on the mat, use a bolster.

■ Bend your knees and place a cushion or rolled-up blanket under your knees.

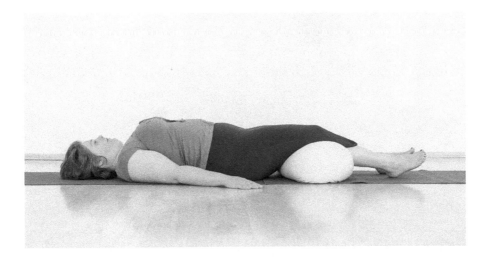

Variation with Bent Knees

As a beginner or if you have a sore back, you may feel uncomfortable with your legs completely stretched out. Here we show you a posture that makes you feel more comfortable and allows you to relax your back.

■ Bend your knees and place your feet flat on the mat, hip width apart.

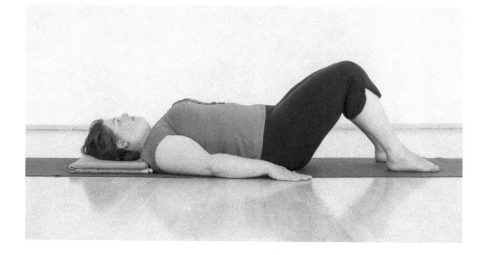

SHANTI ASANA

Purposes

Shanti asana is a supine exercise that enhances your general posture, deepens your breathing, and helps you become focused. The posture is meant to help you become aware of your body, conscious of your breath, and attentive to your thoughts. The more you practice shanti asana, the better you will be able to appraise your actual body tone, your breathing rhythm, and the depth of your breathing. Gradually, you will also become aware of your thoughts and feelings and begin to understand the interplay of asana and feelings.

Notes of Caution and Contraindications

Make sure you do not jump up suddenly. An abrupt jump might lead to a decrease in blood pressure and make you feel dizzy. Inhaling, slowly roll upward into a standing posture or gently move into the next asana. People with high blood pressure or ear or eye conditions should keep their head above heart level by resting it on a cushion or folded blanket while being in shanti asana.

Alignments

In shanti asana, the spinal column is stretched out between your tailbone and the crown of your head. Consciously stretch your neck and lower your chin toward your chest. Relax your shoulder, face, and tongue muscles. Your breath flows in and out through your nose.

Ask yourself the following questions to check for proper alignments and to become more conscious of your whole body:

- Is my neck stretched?
- Is my face relaxed?
- Are my tongue and larynx relaxed?
- Are both my shoulders and both my arms lying evenly on the ground?
- Which parts of my back are in contact with the mat?
- Which parts of my legs and feet are touching the ground?

At the end of a vigorous practice, we recommend that you use a blanket or wear a jacket while being in shanti asana. It is much easier to relax when you feel warm.

What to Do

- Come into the supine starting posture.
- Stretch your entire spine, your legs, and your arms.
- Rotate your feet to the side.
- Put your arms alongside your body with the palms facing the ceiling.
- Relax your shoulders and make sure they are on the mat.
- Stretch your neck and lower your chin toward your sternum.

- Relax your face and mouth muscles.
- Close your eyes. Make sure that you can entirely relax in this position.
- Deeply breathe in and out through your nose.

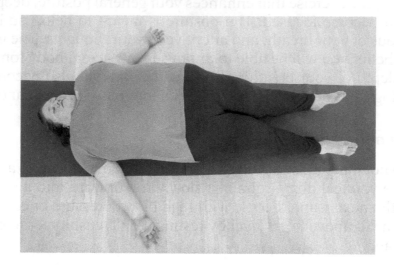

Variation with a Bolster under Your Head

If you are diagnosed with high blood pressure or ear or eye conditions, keep your head above heart level.

- Place your head on a cushion or folded blanket.

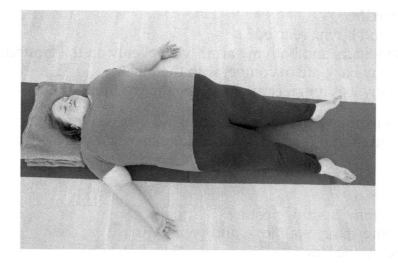

Variation with Bolsters under Your Head and Knees

To relax your back and make the posture more comfortable for you, bend your knees and use a bolster.

■ Place a cushion or rolled-up blanket under your knees.

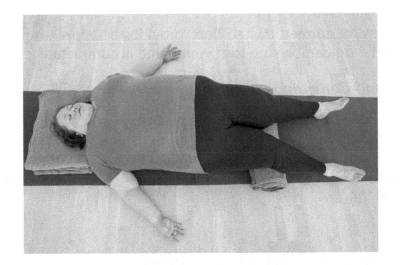

LYING PALM TREE POSTURE

This posture and the tree posture that follows are classically done standing, but, by practicing them on the floor, you will experience the full stretch without worrying about balance. You can find the standing postures further along in this book (see Chapter 11).

Purposes

The palm tree posture performed on the floor provides a secure stretch. If you feel your back against the mat, you can be sure that your spine is completely stretched.

Notes of Caution and Contraindications

There are no general contraindications for this posture. If you suffer from high blood pressure or eye or ear conditions, rest your head on a cushion while performing the posture. Sudden jump-ups out of the postures might lead to decreasing blood pressure and make you feel dizzy. Slowly inhale while rolling upward into a standing posture, or gently move into the following asana.

Alignments

In the palm tree posture, the spinal column is stretched out between pelvis and crown of the head. Feel the stretch in your neck. Your shoulders, your face, and your tongue are relaxed. Your breath flows in and out through the nose.

Notice

You should perform this posture at least two times. Practicing twice allows you to change the way you lace your fingers. Feel the difference between the usual way you lace your fingers and the alternative, with the other thumb in front.

What to Do:

- Come into the supine starting posture.
- Stretch your entire spine, your legs, and your arms.
- Inhaling, lift your arms sideways.
- Lace your fingers and lay your hands on your head with your palms turned outward.

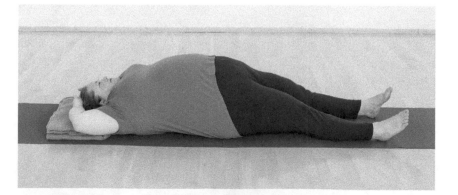

■ Bend your feet. Imagine you are pushing your soles against a wall.

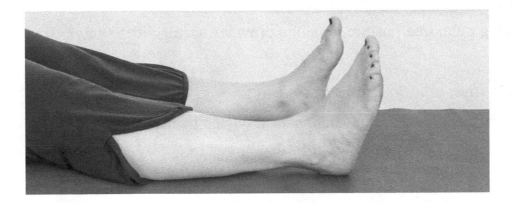

■ Breathe in through your nose while stretching your arms, your back, and your legs.
■ Keep the posture as long as you can comfortably hold your inhalation.

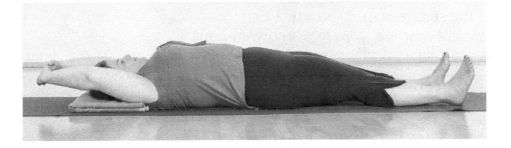

■ Exhaling, get back into the starting position and place your arms sideways.

Second time

■ Lace your hands again. Make sure your other thumb is in front. If it feels strange, you are doing it right.
■ Repeat the movement.
■ Finally, return to the lying posture and feel the effects of the stretch and the deep inhales and exhales. Close your eyes if it feels comfortable.

LYING TREE POSTURE

Purposes

Like the lying palm tree posture, this one provides an excellent stretch. It also opens up your hips.

Notes of Caution and Contraindications

There are no genuine contraindications for the lying tree. Use the same caution that you have used for the lying palm tree posture.

Alignments

The tree posture is meant to enable you to rotate your hip joints fully. Therefore, make sure the outer part of your legs gets in touch with the mat.

What to Do

- Come into the supine starting posture.
- Stretch your entire spine, your legs, and your arms.
- Bend your right leg and place the sole of your right foot against the inner side of your left thigh.

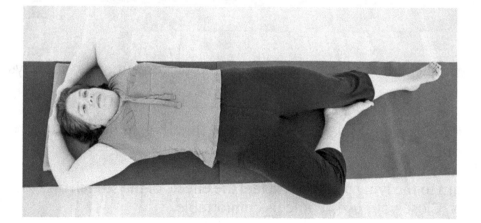

- Your left leg is stretched. Your left foot is bent: your toes point in the direction of your upper body. Make sure that your left sole is flat (think that you are touching a wall with your left sole).

■ Lace your fingers and place your hands on your head (toward your head). Stretch both of your forefingers.

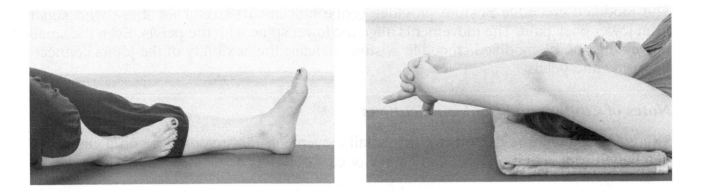

■ Inhaling, stretch your arms, your neck, and your back.
■ Keep the posture for six inhalations and exhalations.
■ Exhaling, get back into the starting position stretching your right leg and lowering your arms sideways.
■ Bend both knees and place your soles hip width apart. Compare the feeling in both sides of your body: both legs, both sides of your pelvis, your shoulders, and your face.
■ Repeat the exercise on the other side and compare the feeling in both sides of your body again. Close your eyes if it feels comfortable.

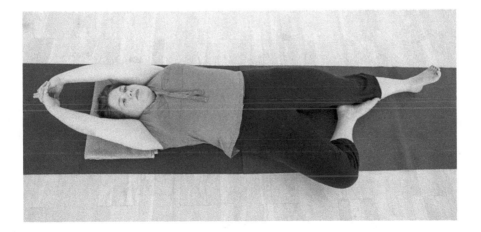

MODIFIED CROCODILE POSTURE

Purposes

The modified crocodile posture provides gentle movements useful for those who suffer from lower back pain. The movements align the lower spine with the pelvis. Even the small movements of the modified crocodile posture increase the flexibility of the joints connecting spine and pelvis.

Notes of Caution and Contraindications

There are no contraindications for this small movement. Place your head on a cushion if you suffer from high blood pressure or eye or ear conditions.

Alignments

Keep your whole spine stretched and in close contact to the mat during the complete movement. Do not forget to stretch your neck and lower your chin toward your chest.

What to Do

- Come into the supine starting posture.
- Stretch your entire spine, your legs, and your arms.
- Place your arms alongside your body with your palms down on the mat.
- Bend your knees and place your feet on the mat. Keep your legs as close together as possible.

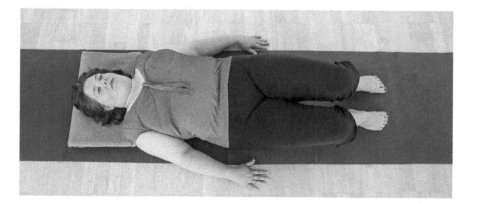

- Exhaling, move your knees and ankles gently to one side. Make sure that you do small movements only a few inches to the side.
- Inhaling, move your knees and ankles back to the center.
- Repeat the side to middle to side movement during at least six complete inhalations and exhalations.

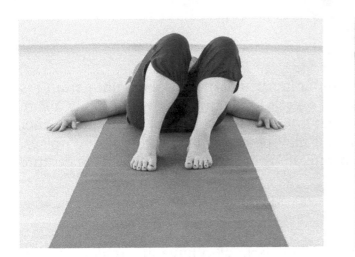
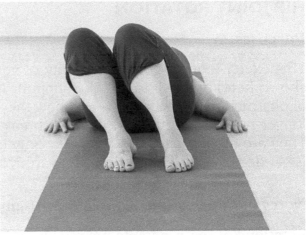

■ Finally, stop the movement, get back into the starting position, and feel the effects of the asana in your lower back.

■ Close your eyes if it feels comfortable.

HIP JOINT ROTATION

Purposes

This exercise enhances the mobility of your hip joints and can be done with a strap (as shown here) or a belt to provide support. If you exercise regularly, you will become aware of obstructions in your joints and how they differ from day to day. In the beginning or after longer periods of sitting or exercise breaks, you may hear popping and cracking noises. They are no cause for concern; they only indicate areas in need of attention. This posture is gentle yet effective for preventing arthrosis.

Notes of Caution and Contraindications

Rotations of the hip joints are strictly forbidden for people who have just undergone hip replacement surgery.

Alignments

Start with small movements, and gradually expand them during the exercise.

Remember to keep your back and neck stretched and lower your chin toward your chest. Rest your head on a cushion or folded blanket if you suffer from high blood pressure or eye or ear conditions.

What to Do

- Come into the supine starting posture.
- Stretch your entire spine, your legs, and your arms.
- Bend your knees and place both your feet hip width apart on the ground.
- Take a strap and place it under your right foot.
- Inhaling, stretch out your right leg. Make sure that your right foot is flexed. (Think of pushing a pedal to accelerate a car.)

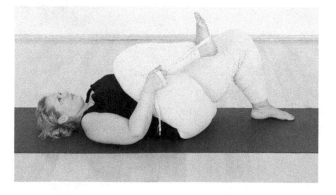 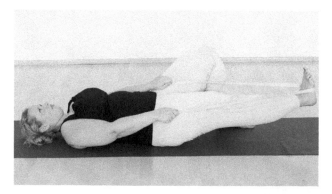

■ In a continuous leg movement, circle to the right. Start with small movements and widen the angle until you move parallel to the floor. Make sure that it feels comfortable.

■ Exhaling, bend your right knee and move it back into the starting position.

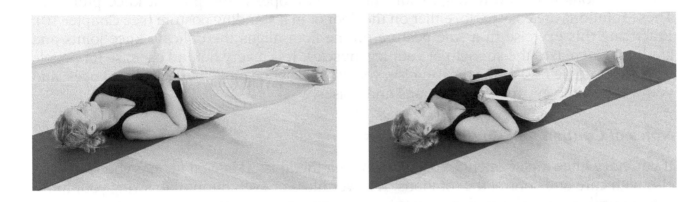

■ Repeat the movement for six complete inhalations and exhalations.

■ Then, still with your right leg, change the direction of the circular movement.

■ Inhaling, rotate your right knee to the right and stretch your right leg. With your right foot flexed, circle your leg to the left in a continuous motion.

■ Exhaling, bend your right leg and move it back into the starting position.

■ Repeat the movement during six complete inhalations and exhalations.

■ Place both feet on the ground and compare the feeling in your right leg and your left leg, in both sides of your pelvis, and in both sides of your face. Feel the polarity of your body, and compare the feeling on the exercising side compared to the other side.

■ Continue with your left leg to the left side.

■ After completing the rotations on the left side, get back into starting position and compare both sides again.

■ Finally, lie on your back and feel the effects of the complete exercise.

SUPINE KNEE ROTATION

Purposes

Knee rotations help you to align your knee joints properly and prevent knee problems. These rotations are easy to do, either on the floor or in a standing posture (see Chapter 10). Practicing this exercise in a safe posture on the floor aligns the delicate knee joints and gradually increases the strength of your leg muscles. It is a very helpful exercise for people with knee problems. During the exercise, you will feel gentle movements in your knees, and you will become aware of obstructions and noises.

Notes of Caution and Contraindications

If you have knee replacements, consult with your therapist. It is vital for everybody to exercise with care and control the rotations. It is worthless or even harmful to swing your lower legs around. Start with small movements and increase them during the exercise.

Alignments

Exercise with slow and controlled movements.

Your spine is stretched, your chin is lowered toward your chest, and, as always, if you suffer from high blood pressure or eye or ear conditions, your head should rest on a cushion or folded blanket.

What to Do

- Come into the supine starting posture.
- Stretch your entire spine, your legs, and your arms.
- Bend your knees and place both your feet hip width apart on the ground.
- Bring your knees closer to your chest, and place your right hand on your right knee and your left hand on your left knee.
- Slowly start moving your lower legs in small circles. As you proceed, feel the movements of your knee joints with your palms. Recognize noises and obstructions.

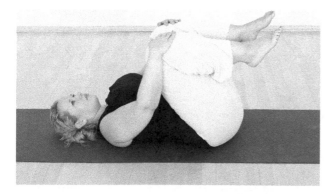 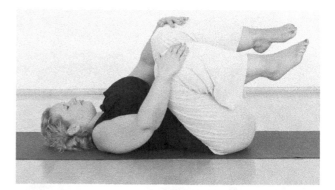

- Synchronize your breathing with your movement (i.e., inhaling during one rotation, exhaling during one rotation).
- Repeat the movements during six complete inhalations and exhalations.
- Continue the exercise rotating in the opposite direction. Notice differences in your knees or differences depending on the direction of the rotation.
- Finally, lie on your back and feel the effects of the complete exercise.

KNEES TO CHEST

Purposes

Knees to chest is an exercise that widens the spaces between the vertebrae. At the same time, the movement deepens your breath. The pressure in your belly rises while you are moving your knees toward your chest. This phase of the movement supports the exhalation. The pressure in the belly lowers while you are moving your knees away from your belly. This phase of the movement supports the inhalation.

It is easy to perform knees to chest. You can even do it while lying in bed (see Chapter 20). This exercise gently stretches your spine, especially the lower back. In the morning, the small but effective movements of this posture can align your vertebrae joints for a better start to the day, and, in the evening, these movements will prepare you for a relaxing sleep.

Notes of Caution and Contraindications

This exercise is very gentle. It can be harmful to someone who suffers from abdominal pain. Use a cushion if you want to keep your head above heart level.

Alignments

It is vital to synchronize your breathing with your movement. Think of exhaling as lowering your abdominal wall and reducing the space of your belly, allowing your knees to come closer to your chest. Think of inhaling as raising your abdominal wall, extending the space and movement, and moving your knees to make space for the belly.

What to Do

■ Come into the supine starting posture.
■ Stretch your entire spine, your legs, and your arms.
■ Bend your knees and place both your feet hip width apart on the ground.
■ Bring your knees closer to your chest, and place your right hand on your right knee and your left hand on your left knee. Make sure that both your lower legs and feet are relaxed and that your neck is stretched.
■ Exhaling, bend your arms and pull your knees closer to your chest.
■ Inhaling, stretch your arms and move your knees away from your chest.
■ Repeat the movement during at least six complete inhalations and exhalations.
■ Place your feet back on the mat and feel the effects of the movement. Close your eyes if it feels comfortable.

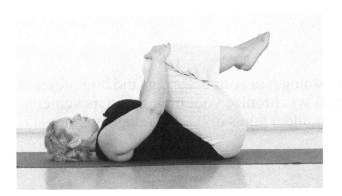
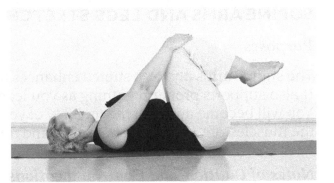

Variation with One Knee at a Time

To make the exercise easier or to allow for the feeling of the polarity of your body, you can exercise with one leg at a time. Use a cushion under your outstretched knee if it feels more comfortable.

What to Do

- Place both feet on the mat.
- You can either stretch your left leg (eventually using a cushion) or keep your left foot on the mat.
- Bring your right knee closer to your chest, and perform knees to chest as demonstrated above.
- Exhaling, reduce the space between belly and thigh.
- Inhaling, extend the space.
- After you have practiced with your right leg, place both feet on the mat, and compare the feeling in both legs, in both sides of your pelvis and both sides of your face. Feel the polarity of your body.
- Now repeat the exercise with your left leg.

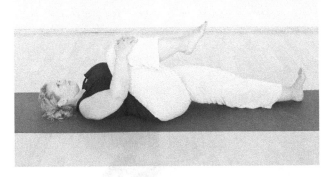
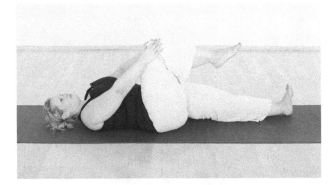

SUPINE ARMS AND LEGS STRETCH

Purposes

The supine arms and legs stretch enhances the strength of your belly, leg, and arm muscles. It also supports proper breathing as you learn to synchronize your breath and movements. You will become aware of the mobility of your shoulder joints and learn to tighten and relax the muscles of your neck, shoulders, and arms.

Notes of Caution and Contraindications

Use a cushion or bolster under your head if you suffer from high blood pressure or ear or eye conditions.

Alignments

Gently stretch your arms and legs when you first start. Recognize the different points of support in both arms and hands lying stretched out on the floor above your head. Regular practice brings you closer to fully stretched out arms and legs and a steady movement.

What to Do

- Come into the supine starting posture.
- Stretch your entire spine, your legs, and your arms.
- Bend your knees and place both your feet hip width apart on the ground.
- Bring your knees closer to your chest. Make sure that both your lower legs and feet are relaxed and that your neck is stretched.
- Place your arms and hands next to your body, palms facing down.
- Inhaling through your nose, lift your arms and stretch your legs upward. The soles of your feet are parallel to the ceiling.

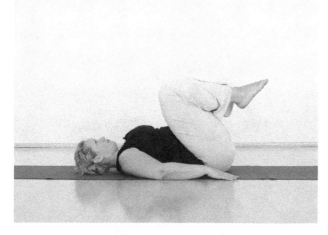
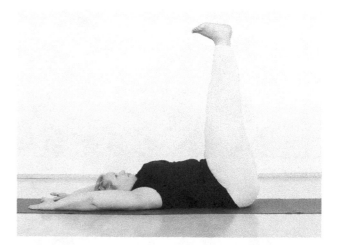

- Exhaling through your nose, lower your arms and bend your legs back into the starting position.
- Repeat the bending and stretching of your legs during six complete inhalations and exhalations.

Part II: Lift Your Stretched Legs

Place your arms stretched out on the mat to the left and right of your body and keep your legs stretched upward to the ceiling.

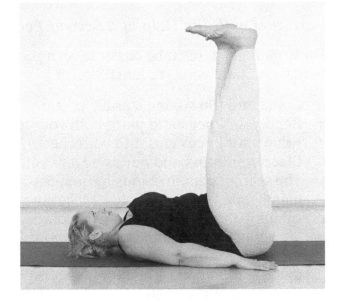

- Alternately lift your right leg and your left leg (keep your feet flexed, soles are parallel to the ceiling). Feel the right and left side of your pelvis lifting from your mat.
- Keep to a steady breathing rhythm that matches the pace of your movements.
- Stop the movement of your legs, and continue with Part III.

Part III: Lift Your Stretched Arms

Keep your legs stretched upward with the soles parallel to the ceiling.

- Inhaling through your nose, lift your arms upward.
- With your arms up and your finger tips pointing to the ceiling, alternate between lifting your right shoulder and your left shoulder up from the mat and lowering it back down.

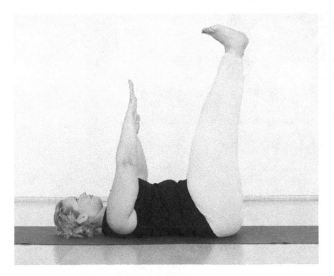

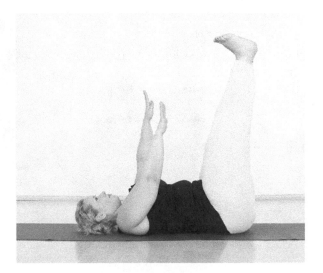

- Keep to a steady breathing rhythm that matches the pace of your movements.
- Stop the movement of your arms.
- Exhaling, lower your arms and legs into the starting position.
- Finally, lie on your back and feel the effects of the exercise. You may close your eyes if you like.

Variation with the Help of a Second Person

For beginners, it might be easier to get a good support, either a yoga teacher or a yogini/yogi (female or male yoga student).

- Come into the supine starting posture.
- Bend your knees and place both your feet hip width apart on the ground.
- Bring your knees closer to your chest.
- Place your arms and hands next to your body, palms facing down.
- The second person stands in front of you in a safe position with her or his feet approximately one leg length apart. Make sure to have eye contact.
- Inhaling through your nose, lift your legs upward.
- Slowly bend your knees and rest your feet on the thighs of the second person. Stay in the posture for six complete inhalation and exhalations. (The second person has to make sure to be in a comfortable position with a stretched back.)
- To get out of the posture place your feet back on the mat one by one.
- Stretch out your legs and feel the effects of the back bow. Close your eyes if it feels comfortable.

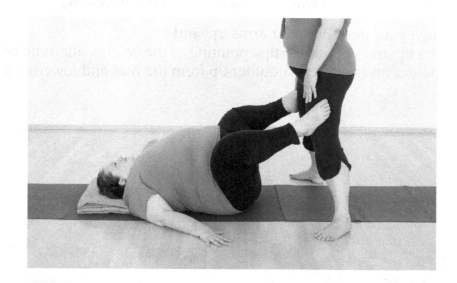

SPIDER POSTURE

Purposes

The spider posture combines stretching and strengthening exercises you have done so far. It provides a vigorous stretch of your spine and legs and also widens the spaces between the vertebrae. At the same time, it challenges your sense of balance.

Notes of Caution and Contraindications

Do not force your legs into an uncomfortable position. It can be harmful to someone who suffers from abdominal pain. Use a cushion to bring your head above heart level if necessary.

Alignments

Keep your feet flexed. To consciously experience the position of your feet, you can start with your hands embracing the forefoot. During the exercise, place your hands under your heels. In both positions, your soles should be parallel to the ceiling. Your thighs should be parallel to the floor. Make sure that your neck is stretched out during the complete time you are exercising.

What to Do

- Come into the supine starting posture.
- Stretch your entire spine, your legs, and your arms.
- Bend your knees and place both feet hip width apart on the ground.
- Bring your knees closer to your chest. Make sure that both your lower legs and feet are relaxed and that your neck is stretched (chin pointing to your chest).

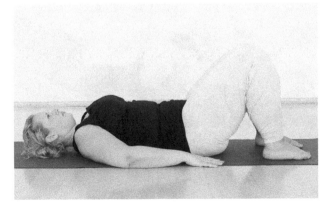 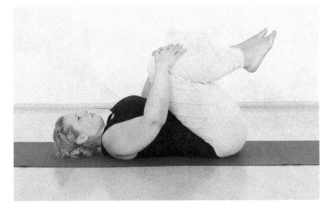

- Bring your arms between your knees and hold your right foot with your right hand and your left foot with your left hand. Make sure your feet are bent and your soles are parallel to the floor.
- Move your hands to get hold of your heels. Make sure your neck is still stretched and your chin is pointing to your chest.
- Exhaling through your nose, slowly swing your body to your left side.
- Inhaling through your nose, slowly swing your body to the right side.
- Repeat the movement for six complete inhalations and exhalations.
- Lower your legs and arms. Place your feet on your mat and your arms at the side of your body.
- Feel the effects of the movement. Close your eyes if it feels comfortable for you.

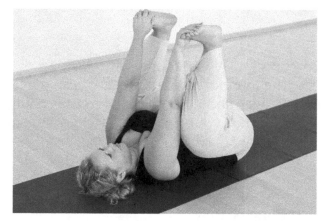

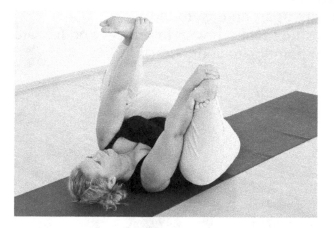

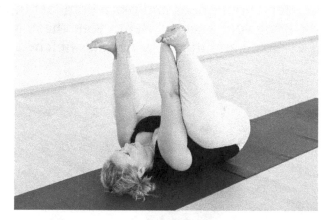

SHOULDER BRIDGE

Purposes

The shoulder bridge enhances the mobility of your spine and the strength of your leg and back muscles. It can be done either in motion or as a posture. Alternately bowing and stretching your spine improves the mobility of the vertebrae while keeping your spine in a backward bend increases the strength of your leg and back muscles.

Notes of Caution and Contraindications

This exercise can be harmful if you have high blood pressure or if you suffer from eye or ear conditions.

Alignments

Make sure that your neck is stretched out during the complete time you are exercising. Do not bend your neck while you are raising your spine. Keep your knees parallel and hip width apart. Push your soles completely into your mat; do not shift your weight either to the inner or outer sides of your feet.

What to Do

In Motion

- Come into the supine starting posture.
- Stretch your entire spine, your legs, and your arms.
- Bend your knees and place both feet hip width apart on the ground.
- Place your arms on the mat next to your sides. Your palms are facing downward.
- During a complete inhalation, tighten your bottom or, better, your pelvic muscles, and lift your back vertebra by vertebra.

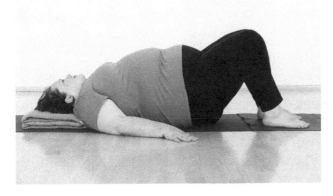 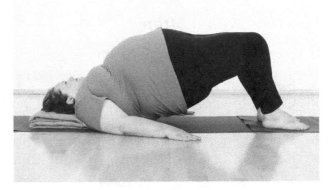

- During a complete exhalation, lower your back vertebra by vertebra. Relax your pelvic muscles at the end of the movement.
- Make sure your breathing and moving are completely synchronized.
- Repeat the movements for six complete inhalations and exhalations.

Posture

- To do the asana, check the position of your neck, feet, and knees, and lift your vertebrae once again during an inhalation.
- With the next inhalation, lift both your arms and place them on the mat above your head.

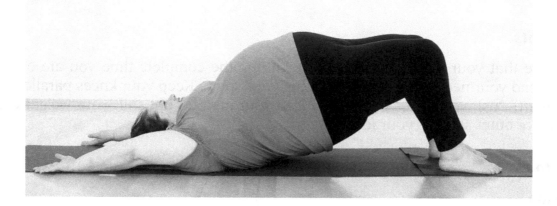

- Keep the posture for six complete inhalations and exhalations. Make sure that your spine is in the form of a bridge. Get as much space between your upper spine and the mat as possible—without hurting yourself.
- To get out of the posture, lower your spine vertebra by vertebra as well as your arms during a complete exhalation.
- Stretch out your legs and feel the effects of the back bend. Close your eyes if it feels comfortable.

Variation with a Strap

If you want to make sure to stay aligned, use a strap or belt.

- Start stretched out on your back.
- Check the position of your neck, feet, and knees once again; lift your vertebrae and stay in the asana.
- Place a strap around your lower legs above your ankles.
- Keep both ends of the strap in your hands, and extend the back bow with an inhalation.

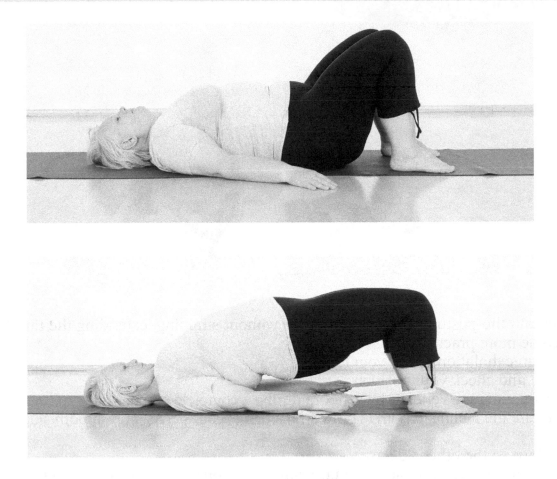

- To get out of the posture, remove the strap.
- Lower your spine vertebra by vertebra during a complete exhalation.
- Stretch out your legs and feel the effects of the back bow. Close your eyes if it feels comfortable.

Variation with an Outstretched Leg

If it is easy for you to stay aligned, stretch one leg at a time and lift it.

- Start in the shoulder bridge posture.
- Check the position of your neck, feet, and knees once again.
- With an inhalation, lift your right leg.

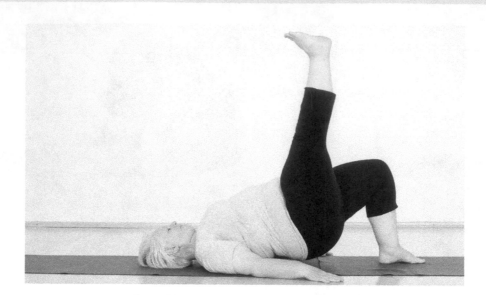

- Maintain the posture as long as you can without straining, extending the time as you become more practiced.
- With an exhalation, lower your leg.
- Inhale and check your position.
- Lower your spine vertebra by vertebra during a complete exhalation.
- Compare the feeling in both legs, in both sides of your pelvis, and in both sides of your face.
- Continue to the other side.
- At the end of the complete asana, stretch out your legs, and feel the effects of the intense back bow. Close your eyes if it feels comfortable.

4

Postures Lying on the Side

Like the supine postures, these postures realign vertebrae and joints and are performed while you are stretched out on the floor. However, it is much harder to maintain alignment when lying on your side. Be sure not to bend forward or backward. A much smaller range of motion is possible while you are lying on your side; keep to the smaller movements and stay aligned.

LEG LIFT SIDEWAYS

Purposes

This sideways-bending posture mobilizes hip joints and enhances the flexibility and strength of your inner and outer hip and leg muscles. It also increases breathing capacity. While you are lying on your side, both of your nostrils sink, leading to the narrowing of your upper and widening of your lower nasal cavity. The effects are comparable to those of the alternate nostril breathing (see p. 160). This exercise can be done in motion or as a posture. It is most effective if you exercise both ways.

Notes of Caution and Contraindications

Bend your lower arm and rest your head in your palm if you are diagnosed with high blood pressure or if you suffer from eye or ear conditions. This way, your head will remain above heart level.

Alignments

Make sure that your body and legs are fully stretched out during the whole time that you are exercising. Tighten your pelvic muscles and avoid bending your torso. Do not rotate your exercising leg. It is easier for the exercise in motion as well as for the posture if you push your lower leg against the floor while you are lifting your upper leg.

What to Do

- Stretch out on your back.
- Stretch your neck with your chin pointing toward your chest.
- Stretch your back and your legs. Tighten your bottom muscles. Flex your feet so that your toes point toward the ceiling.
- Inhaling, stretch your right arm, lift it upward, and rest it on the floor above your head.
- Exhaling, turn your body and legs to the right side. Rest your head on your right arm. (If it is more comfortable for you or if you suffer from high blood pressure or eye or ear conditions, bend your right arm and place your head into your right palm.)
- To stabilize your position, place your left hand flat on the mat in front of you. Your fingers are pointing into the direction of your head. Make sure that your body is fully stretched out and that you are not bending your upper body. Your feet are bent, with toes and feet pulled toward your belly.

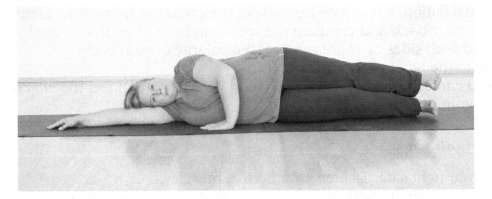

- Relax your face, lips, and tongue muscles.
- Breathe in and out deeply through your nose.
- Inhaling, lift your upper leg. Make sure you are moving slowly, synchronizing breathing and movement. Lift your leg without rotating your foot (the heel is leading the movement).

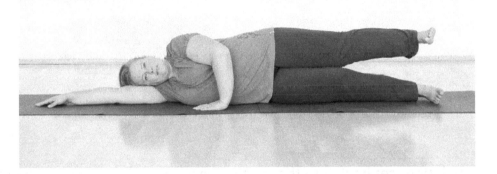

- Exhaling, lower your upper leg.
- Repeat the movement during six full inhalations and exhalations.
- After an inhalation, stay in the posture for six complete inhalations and exhalations.

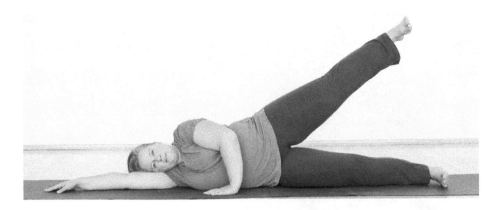

- With an exhalation, lower your leg and get back into the starting position.
- Turn onto your back and compare the feeling in both of your legs, both sides of your pelvis, and both sides of your face. Feel the polarity of your body.
- Continue to the other side.
- Either you can complete the exercise, lie on your back, and feel the effects of the exercise, or continue with Part II.

Part II: Lift Both Legs

- Start on your right side. Tighten your bottom muscles.
- With an inhalation, lift both legs. Make sure that you do not bend your body or lift your legs forward. The sideway lift of both legs can only be a small movement.
- With an exhalation, lower both legs.
- Continue the lifting and lowering with a synchronized breath.
- After moving into and out of the posture, keep the posture with both legs lifted.

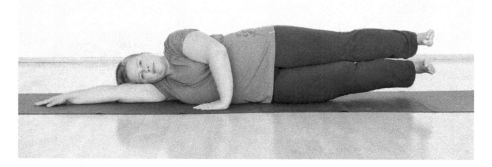

- With an exhalation, get back into the starting position and compare both sides.
- Continue to the other side.
- Finally, lie on your back and feel the effects of the complete exercise.

HEAD LIFT SIDEWAYS

Purposes

Bending your head to the side mobilizes the joints of your cervical vertebrae and enhances the flexibility of the blood vessels and muscles of your neck. This exercise mobilizes your upper spine and can be done in motion or as a posture.

Notes of Caution and Contraindications

This exercise is not recommended if you suffer from serious neck pain or are diagnosed with high blood pressure or suffer from eye or ear conditions.

Alignments

Make sure that your spine is fully stretched. Do not rotate your head.

What to Do

- Come into the dorsal starting posture.
- Stretch your neck with your chin pointing toward your chest.
- Stretch your back and your legs. Tighten your bottom muscles. Flex your feet so that your toes point toward the ceiling.
- Inhaling, stretch your right arm, lift it upward, and rest it on the floor above your head.
- Exhaling, turn your body and legs to the right side. Rest your head on your right arm.
- To stabilize your position, place your left hand flat on the mat in front of your sternum with the fingers pointed in the direction of your head. Make sure that your body is fully stretched out and that you are not bending your upper body. Your feet are bent: your feet and toes are pointing toward your belly.
- Relax your face, lips, and tongue muscles.
- Breathe in and out deeply through your nose.
- Inhaling, lift your head. Make sure that you do not rotate your head.

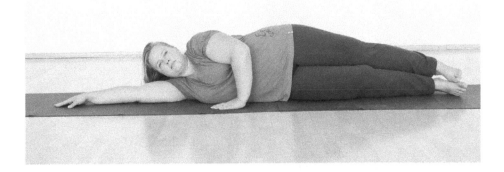

- Exhaling, lower your head.
- Repeat the movement during six full inhalations and exhalations.
- Turn onto your back, and compare the feeling in both sides of your head and both sides of your face.
- Continue to the other side.
- Finally, lie on your back and feel the effects of the complete exercise.

5

Postures Lying on the Stomach (Prone)

The following exercises and postures realign vertebrae and joints in a backward bend. They also use the floor as a prop. At the beginning of your yoga practice, you may find lying on your belly (prone posture) challenging. Leg lifts, for example, seem to be more difficult in this position. Breathing will also feel different while you lie on your stomach, as different parts of the lungs are ventilated while you exercise in this position.

For best results, start with small movements and extend them slowly. Tighten the pelvic muscles and be easy with the backbends, especially if you have problems with your lower back. It is better to stretch and gain length than to bend and get hurt.

PRONE ARMS AND LEGS STRETCH

Purposes

The prone arms and legs stretch is an exercise that is very efficient for building muscles and improving back flexibility. These improvements are especially valuable for people who work in a seated posture (i.e., in front of a computer, at a desk). Working in a seated and forward bowing position can lead to a rounded upper back. Stretches of the entire spine in a backward bend can counteract the poor posture.

Notes of Caution and Contraindications

The pressure on the belly vessels may increase blood pressure. Therefore, it is important for people with high blood pressure or eye or ear conditions to do the ventral posture with caution. People with serious problems in their lower back have to tighten the pelvic muscles during the whole exercise and take it easy with the backbend. It is better for them to stretch and gain length than to bend and get hurt.

Alignments

It is vital to fully stretch out the spinal column and tighten the pelvic muscles. Arms, legs, and the complete spine—including the neck—should be lengthened. Look down to your mat while lifting your head. Make sure your heels do not rotate.

What to Do

- Stretch out lying on your belly.
- Place your forehead on your mat.

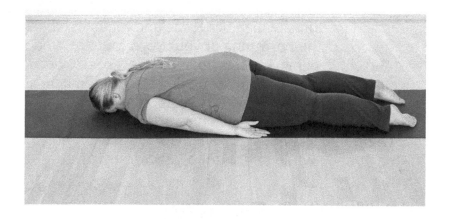

- Inhaling, stretch out both arms and both legs.
- Tighten your bottom muscles (better: tighten your pelvic muscles). Keep these muscles tight during the whole asana.

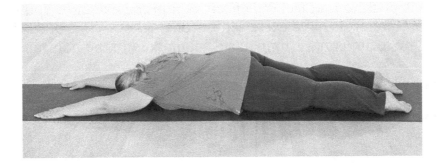

- Inhaling, lengthen your right arm and left leg and slowly lift them together with your head. Make sure you are looking downward with your neck stretched out.

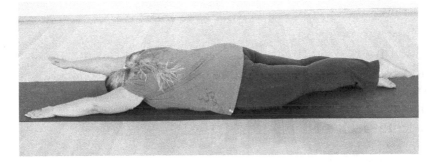

- Exhaling, lower your arm, leg, and head into the starting position.
- Inhaling, lengthen your left arm and right leg and slowly lift them together with your head. Make sure that you are looking downward with your neck stretched out.
- Repeat the movement alternating the sides.
- Keep to a steady breathing rhythm that matches the pace of your movements for at least six full inhalations and exhalations.
- Finally, turn onto your back again and feel the effects of the whole exercise. Close your eyes if it feels more comfortable.

PRONE SHANTI ASANA

Purposes

The prone shanti asana is a relaxing posture to do between exercises or after exercising. You can rest in this posture and feel the effects of a prone exercise. You can also use the posture as a break after you have exercised on one side of your body. It allows you to become aware of the feeling on the trained side compared to the nontrained side.

Notes of Caution and Contraindications

There are no general contraindications. Exercise with care.

Alignments

Relax your body. Rest your head on one side (change sides if you take several rests). Your palms are facing upward toward the ceiling. Your heels are rotated to the outside.

What to Do

- Stretch out in a prone position.
- Place to the side and rest on the right ear. Forehead on the mat, with your arms beside your body and your legs and feet stretched out.
- Exhaling, turn your head to the left side and rest on your right ear. Inhaling, find a relaxed position for your head.
- Exhaling, turn your heels outward.

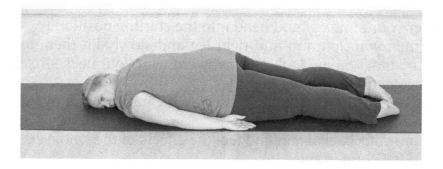

- Turn your head to the side and rest on your left ear, when taking another break.

SPHINX POSTURE

Purposes

The sphinx posture is a gentle backbend for the spine with the support of your forearms. This posture lengthens the front side of your hip and thigh muscles and mobilizes the spine.

Notes of Caution and Contraindications

If you suffer from serious problems in your lower back, make sure that you keep your pelvic muscles tight and be easy with the backbend. Think of stretching and lengthening your spine, and do not force your torso into a backbend and get hurt.

Alignments

Your elbows are under your shoulder joints. Keep your neck stretched and your shoulders down while lifting your head and trunk.

What to Do

- Stretch out in a prone position.
- Place your forehead on your mat, with your legs and feet stretched out.
- Bend both arms and place your hands next to your shoulders.
- Tighten your bottom muscles (better: tighten your pelvic muscles). Keep these muscles tight during the whole posture.
- Inhaling, lengthen your spine and slowly lift your head and trunk. Make sure that your neck is stretched out.
- Place your forearms on the mat to come into the sphinx posture. Make sure your elbows are in line with your shoulders. Keep your neck stretched and your shoulders down.

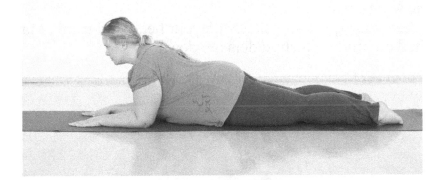

- Stay in the sphinx posture for six complete inhalations and exhalations.
- Exhaling, slowly lower your head and trunk.
- Feel the effects in the prone shanti asana postur, or turn onto your back and rest in the supine shanti posture. Close your eyes if it feels comfortable.

COBRA POSTURE

Purposes

The cobra posture is a stronger backbend for the spine with more weight on your forearms. It provides an intense lengthening of the front side of your hip and thigh muscles, and it vigorously mobilizes the spine.

> *"Cobra posture and free seats are my favorite postures. I can do both very well."*
> —Doris

Notes of Caution and Contraindications

If you suffer from serious problems in your lower back, you should stay in the sphinx posture and build muscles before going into the cobra posture. Keep your pelvic muscles tight, and do not force your trunk into a backbend.

Alignments

It is vital to fully stretch out the spinal column and tighten the pelvic muscles. Arms, legs, and the complete spine—including the neck—should be lengthened. Make sure that you do not block your elbow joints.

What to Do

- Stretch out in a prone position.
- Place your forehead on the mat, with your legs and feet stretched out.
- Bend both arms and place your hands next to your shoulders.
- Tighten your bottom muscles (better: tighten your pelvic muscles). Keep these muscles tight during the whole asana.
- Inhaling, lengthen your spine and slowly lift your head and trunk. Make sure that your neck is stretched out and your shoulders are down.

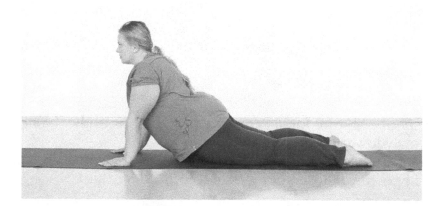

- Exhaling, slowly lower your head and trunk. Synchronize your breath with your movements.
- You can either lift and lower your head and torso in your breath rhythm, or stay in the cobra posture for a couple of complete inhalations and exhalations. (Take a break if necessary.)
- Feel the effects in the prone shanti asana, or turn onto your back and rest in the supine shanti asana. Close your eyes if you like to do so.

Variation with the Help of a Second Person

If you are an experienced yogini/yogi, it can be helpful to get an extra stretch with the help of a friend.

- Start in a prone position with your forehead on the mat and your arms at the side.
- Ask a fellow student to sit between your feet on your mat and take your wrists while you take her or his wrists. Make sure that the position works well for both of you.
- With an inhalation, the lying person lifts the torso while at the same time with an inhalation the sitting person carefully pulls the arms of the lying person backward.

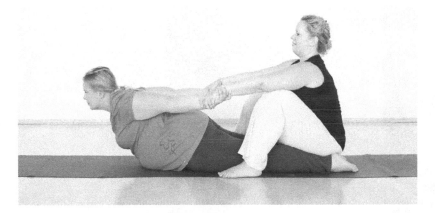

- With both of you exhaling, lower the torso.
- Feel the effects in the prone shanti asana, or turn onto your back and rest in the supine shanti asana. Close your eyes if it feels comfortable.

Variation with a Wall

This variation of the cobra posture gives you a gentle stretch of the front side of your hip and thigh muscles. It mobilizes your vertebrae without hurting your lower back. It can also be done during the day if you need a stretch and backbend.

- Stand upright facing a wall.
- Place your feet hip width apart on the floor and your palms on the wall at the height of your shoulders.
- Step forward until the tips of your toes, your belly, your forearms, and your forehead are in contact with the wall. Tighten your pelvic muscles and stretch your spine—including your neck.
- Inhaling, slowly bend your head and upper spine backward. Pause and stretch your spine again. Inhaling, gently enlarge your back bow. Your toes, belly, and forearms keep in touch with the wall while you are bending your trunk and head backward.

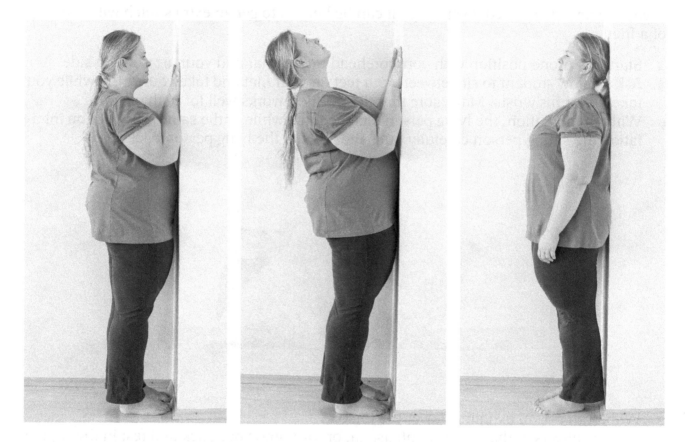

- Stay in a comfortable posture for about six inhalations and exhalations.
- With an exhalation, slowly return to the starting posture.
- Turn around and lean with your back against the wall.
- Feel the effect of the exercise.

LYING BOW POSTURE

Purposes

This posture is an intense backward bend that enhances the mobility of your spine. It is especially challenging to the muscles on the front of your hips and thighs. With the backward bend of your spine and arms, the breathing space widens and allows deeper inhalations and exhalations. Here we are demonstrating the posture with a strap or belt as a prop.

Notes of Caution and Contraindications

If you suffer from serious problems in your lower back, you should not perform the lying bow posture.

Alignments

Keep your knees hip width apart during the whole exercise. Make sure your spinal column is fully stretched out before you bend backward. Keep your pelvic muscles tight and relax your shoulders.

What to Do

- Stretch out in a prone position.
- Place your forehead on your mat, with your arms beside your body and your legs and feet stretched out.
- Tighten your pelvic muscles and keep them tight during the whole asana.
- Bend your knees and place a strap around your ankles (ask someone for assistance if necessary). Hold the ends of the strap with both your hands.

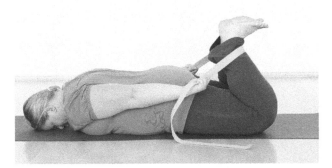 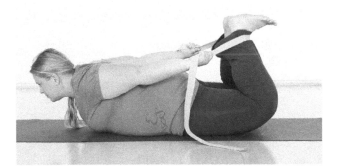

- Stretch your spine again in this position with your forehead still on the mat.
- With an inhalation, lift your torso and your thighs with the help of the strap. Pause on an exhale.
- With an inhalation, extend the backbend.
- Keep the position for six complete inhalations and exhalations.
- Exhaling, slowly lower your head, legs, and arms. Turn your head to the side and rest your head on one ear. Place your arms at the side with your palms facing upward. Let both heels glide to the sides (prone shanti asana).
- Rest in this posture and feel the effects of the strong backbend.

6

Seated Postures and Bows

It takes practice to be able to sit upright on a mat with legs outstretched, so in this chapter we provide variations with bolsters and bent knees. To get the most out of your practice, start by choosing the upright seated posture that works best for you. Experiment with the recommended variations, and do not hesitate to use a prop if it helps you feel comfortable. Always remember: yoga is bhoga (joy).

STAFF POSTURE

Purposes

The staff posture is the starting position for many yoga exercises. Although it is easy to understand, it is hard to master. We are used to sitting on chairs and sofas with our knees bent. An upright seated position with unbent knees and outstretched legs is uncommon to us. This posture and its variations are very helpful to build muscles that keep the pelvis in an upright position. In the staff posture, you also stretch the muscles on the back of your thighs.

Notes of Caution and Contraindications

There are no general contraindications to the staff posture. However, there are some ways in which it can be made easier. As always, exercise with care and be gentle to your body.

Alignments

The spinal column is stretched out from your sit bones (the bones under your buttocks) to the crown of your head. Feel the stretch in your neck. Your chin is parallel to the ground, and your shoulders and arms, as well as your face and tongue muscles, are relaxed. Your breath flows slowly in and out through your nose.

What to Do

- Sit on the mat and distribute your weight evenly on both sit bones.
- Position your feet hip width apart.
- Flex your feet and pull your toes in the direction of your belly.
- Your pelvis is upright, your spinal column is stretched, and the crown of your head extends upward.
- Your sternum is raised, and your hands lie loosely on your thighs.
- Your chin is parallel to the ground, and your face, lips, and tongue are relaxed.
- Breathe in and out deeply through your nose.

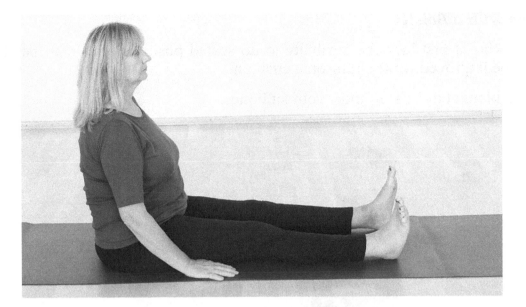

■ Keep the posture during six complete inhalations and exhalations.

Variation with Hands on the Mat

If you cannot stretch your spine during six complete inhalations and exhalations, try the following variation:

■ Place both hands behind your back on the floor on either side of your pelvis to support your proper alignment.

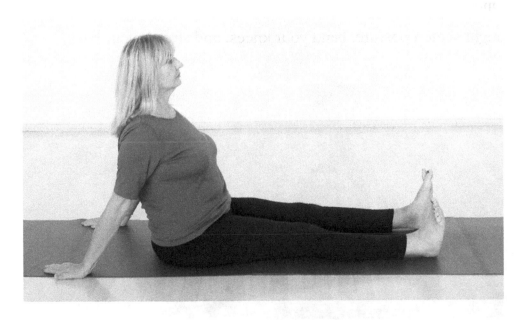

Variation with a Bolster

For those who at first lack the flexibility to do seated postures on a mat, flexibility can gradually be improved while sitting on a cushion.

■ Place a blanket or bolster under your sit bones.

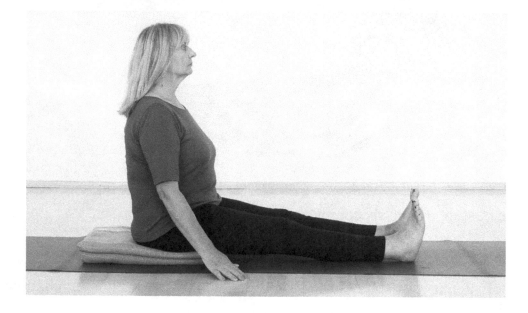

Variation with Crossed Legs

Some of the seated yoga postures can be performed with bent knees to keep the spine properly aligned.

■ Sit in upright seated posture, bend your knees, and stretch your back.

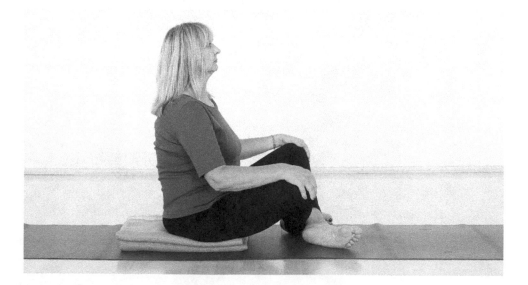

SEATED POSTURE ON A CHAIR

Purposes

Sitting upright on a chair is a good practice to feel the proper alignment of your spine. Occasionally during the day, while sitting in a car or at a desk, check on your seated posture. This is the correct posture to start yoga exercises if you have trouble sitting upright on your mat.

Notes of Caution and Contraindications

There are no general contraindications.

Alignments

Place your knees over your ankles. Stretch your spine and keep your pelvis in an upright position. Your chin is parallel to the ground, and your shoulders and arms, as well as your face and tongue muscles, are relaxed.

What to Do

■ Sit on a chair and distribute your weight evenly on both sit bones (buttocks).
■ Position your feet hip width apart. The weight of your legs should be evenly distributed on your feet. The outer edges of your feet are parallel to one another.
■ Your knee joints are directly above your ankles.
■ Your pelvis is upright, your spinal column is stretched, and the crown of your head extends upward.
■ Your sternum is raised, and your hands lie loosely on your thighs.
■ Your chin is parallel to the ground, and your face, lips, and tongue are relaxed.
■ Breathe in and out deeply through your nose.
■ Keep the posture during six complete inhalations and exhalations.

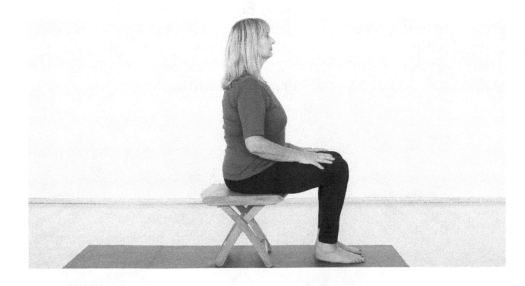

HEAD TO KNEE

Purposes

Head to knee is a forward bow. It stretches the muscles of the back of your legs and your pelvis as well as your back muscles. Beginners often focus on the wrong priority: Can I touch my toes? They forget about the most important part of the exercise: Is my spine fully stretched out? A forward bend without stretching the vertebrae is a reason for backaches—in everyday life as well as in doing yoga.

Forward bends are very common movements in daily life and are often accompanied by back pains. Underdeveloped muscles in the back (interacting with the belly muscles) are the reason for poor pelvic alignment. The pelvis is tilted forward, and the spine is slightly bent forward in its lower part and often rounded in its upper part. This poor posture is a serious hardship. Yoga helps you to develop a proper position and keep you upright without feeling unnatural.

Notes of Caution and Contraindications

This posture is not recommended if you have acute back or stomach pain.

Alignments

It is vital to stretch the vertebrae from your sit bones to the crown of your head during the whole asana. Use a bolster, and practice a variation if it helps you to stay aligned. These variations are helpful because they allow a proper stretch without reducing the intensity of the forward bend.

What to Do

- Come into staff posture.
- Make sure your feet are hip width apart and flexed, your pelvis is upright, your spinal column is stretched, and the crown of your head extends upward.
- Place a strap around your feet.
- Inhaling, stretch your torso.
- Exhaling, bend your upper torso forward. Make sure that your spine is always stretched (including the neck; do not bow your head backward).

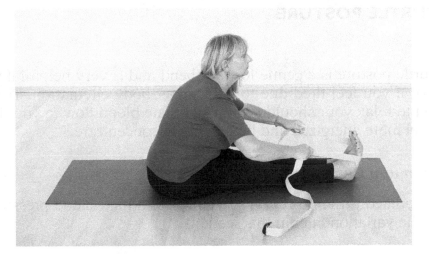

- Inhaling, stretch your torso again.
- Exhaling, lower your trunk again if you want to intensify the forward bow.
- Keep your position for six complete inhalations and exhalations.
- To get back into starting position: Inhaling, slowly raise your trunk, head, and arms.
- Exhaling, rest your arms in your lap.
- Either stay in the upright posture or stretch out on the floor to feel the effects of the exercise in the back of your legs, your torso, and your pelvis.

Variations with a Bolster under Your Buttocks

In the beginning, the muscles gain more flexibility if you reduce the stretch.

- Place a bolster under your buttocks before getting into the upright seated posture, and continue as described earlier.

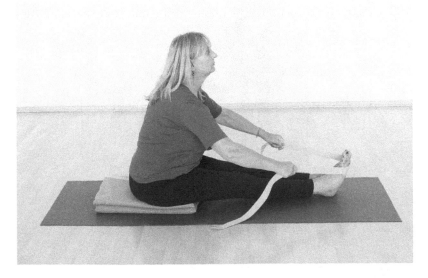

MODIFIED TURTLE POSTURE

Purposes

The modified turtle posture is a gentle forward bend and is very helpful if you suffer from stiff shoulders or if you feel tired due to poor upper body circulation. This easy forward bend allows you to relax your shoulders and stimulate blood flow to your head, ears, and eyes. You will feel more energized and better able to concentrate.

Notes of Caution and Contraindications

Do not do the modified turtle posture if you suffer from high blood pressure or eye or ear conditions (see the variation later in this section).

Alignments

Keep your spine stretched out and relax your shoulder and arms as well as your face and tongue muscles. Your knees and ankles are in one line.

What to Do

- Come into the upright seated posture on a chair.
- Place your feet more than hip width apart.
- Make sure your knee joints are directly above your ankles, your pelvis is upright, your spinal column is stretched, and the crown of your head extends upward.
- Your shoulders and arms are relaxed as well as your face and tongue muscles.

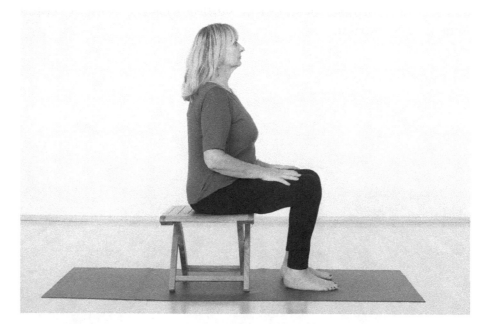

- Inhaling, stretch your spine.
- Exhaling bend downward between your knees, placing your hands around your lower legs or ankles. Relax your neck muscles.

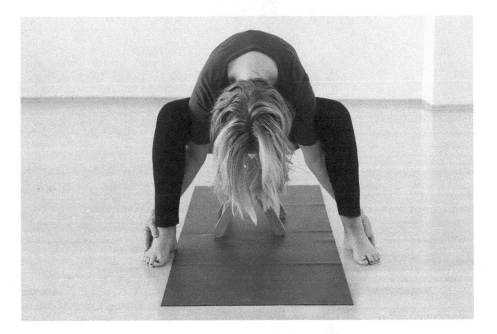

- Maintain the position for six complete inhalations and exhalations. With each exhalation, relax your shoulders. With each inhalation, feel the stretch of your spine.
- To get out of the posture: Inhaling, raise your stretched spine into the starting position.
- Sit in an upright position and feel the effects of the exercise in your head and shoulders. Keep your eyes closed if it feels comfortable.

Variation with Arms on the Knees

If you want to relax your arms and shoulders and get a gentle stretch in your lower back without lowering your head under heart level, try the following variation.

- Come into the upright seated posture on a chair.
- Place your feet more than hip width apart.
- Make sure that your knee joints are directly above your ankles, your pelvis is upright, your spinal column is stretched, and the crown of your head extends upward.
- Your shoulders and arms are relaxed as well as your face and tongue muscles.
- Inhaling, stretch your spine.
- Exhaling, lower your torso and place your forearms on top of your thighs.

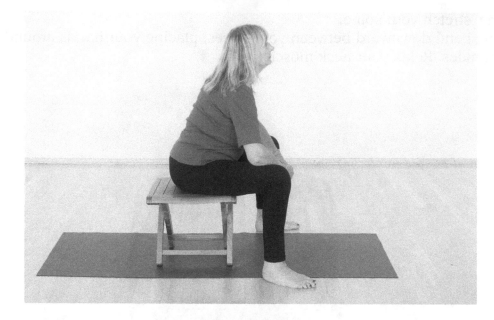

■ Keep the posture for six complete inhalations and exhalations.

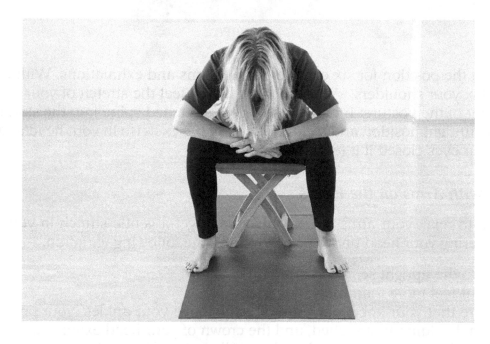

■ To get out of the posture: Inhaling, raise your stretched spine into the starting position.
■ Sit in an upright position and feel the effects of the exercise in your head and shoulders. Keep your eyes closed if it feels comfortable.

HEAD BOW SIDEWAYS

Purposes

The bow of your head is very helpful to stretch your neck muscles and enhance the blood circulation. It is also a good remedy if you suffer from stiff shoulders. This easy move stretches your neck muscles in one direction and helps you to prevent a stiff neck or stiff shoulders, which can lead to headaches. Even if your neck and shoulders already hurt or if you have problems moving your head, this little exercise is a good start to regain a normal mobility.

Notes of Caution and Contraindications

A warm shawl or a heating pad can support mobility and help you to get back into motion. To control the movement better, it is important that you do not bow and rotate your head at the same time.

Alignments

Keep your spine stretched out and relax your shoulders. Close your eyes if it helps you to concentrate better and feel the effects of this small but valuable exercise.

- Come into upright seated posture on a chair.
- Place your feet hip width apart.
- Inhaling, stretch your spine and relax your shoulders. Keep your chin parallel to the floor to maximize the stretch of your neck.

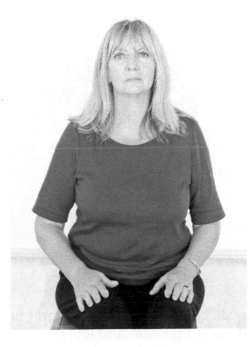

- Exhaling, gently bow your head to the side—bring your left ear closer to your left shoulder. Make sure that both your shoulders stay relaxed.

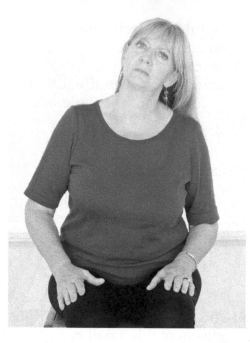

- Inhaling again, get back into the starting position and stretch your spine again.
- Exhaling, gently bow your head to the side—bring your right ear closer to your right shoulder. Make sure that both your shoulders stay relaxed.

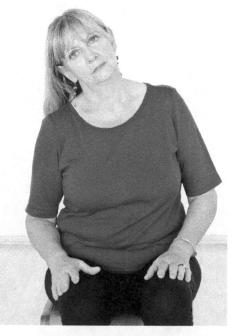

- Repeat the movements for six complete inhalations and exhalations.
- Finally, stay in the upright seated posture and feel the effects of the exercise.

FISH POSTURE

Purposes

The fish posture is a strong and very effective backbend. It stretches the rib cage and enlarges the breathing space. At the same time, it mobilizes the spine—especially the neck—as well as the shoulders.

During daily life, backward bends are rare. Our most common movement is a forward bend. When we are sitting or standing, we work with our hands; we look down and we bend forward. As a result, a humpback is often noticeable. Many of us also tend to rush around and do a lot of things at the same time. Our posture as well as our attitude is often a forward motion—to get things done. In profile, we often look like question marks. It is good for us to slowly bend our upper torso backward and to realign. This strong backward bend counteracts a humpback and expands breathing capacity.

Notes of Caution and Contraindications

If you suffer from high blood pressure or eye or ear conditions, it is better to do a backward bend in a standing posture. If you feel sick bowing your head backward, return to the starting posture.

Alignments

Relax your shoulders and keep your elbows in line with your shoulder joints. Your legs are fully stretched out and hip width apart.

What to Do

- Sit on the mat and distribute your weight evenly on both sit bones.
- Your pelvis is upright, your spinal column is stretched, and the crown of your head extends upward.
- Place both hands behind your back on the floor on either side of your pelvis with your fingers pointing toward your back.
- Position your feet hip width apart. Flex your feet and pull your toes in the direction of your belly.
- Your chin is parallel to the ground and your face, lips, and tongue are relaxed.
- Breathe in and out deeply through your nose.

■ Exhaling, slowly lower your torso and bend your arms until your forearms are on the mat. Make sure that your elbows are underneath your shoulder joints.

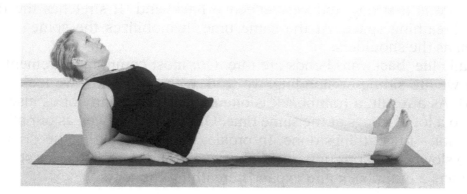

■ Inhaling, bend your upper torso backward until the crown of your head touches the ground.
■ Place your hands on top of your belly near the groin. Lift your rib cage, keeping your pelvis on the ground.

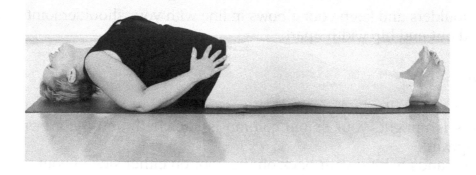

■ Keep the position for six complete inhalations and exhalations.
■ With an exhalation, move your elbows and arms to the side and lower your torso. Stretch out on your mat.
■ Feel the effects of the backward bend in your upper torso. Close your eyes if it feels comfortable.

MODIFIED TABLE POSTURE

Purposes

The table posture strengthens arm, leg, belly, and back muscles. We demonstrate the modified version with a bench as prop. In the modified version, you start sitting on a bench and move downward. This way you get the same benefits without the strain of lifting your body with a hard push.

Notes of Caution and Contraindications

Make sure that the chair or bench is securely anchored. Get a good grip of the prop. Keep your head above heart level, if necessary.

Alignments

Place your ankles under your knees and your wrist under your shoulders to be gentle to your joints. Do not lock your elbows.

What to Do

- Come into the seated posture on a securely anchored bench or chair.
- Place your feet hip joint width apart. Your ankles are under your knees.
- Place your hands behind your back either on top of the bench or grasp the edge.

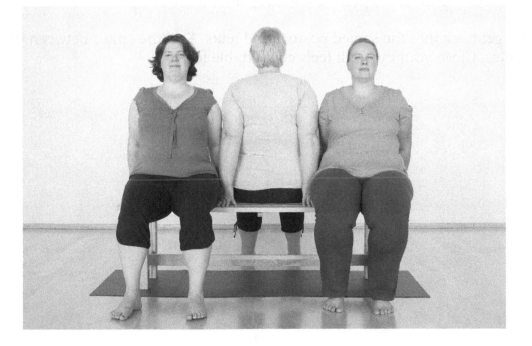

- Inhaling, tighten your pelvic muscles and lift your body.

■ Make sure your hands are underneath your shoulders and your ankles are underneath your knees.

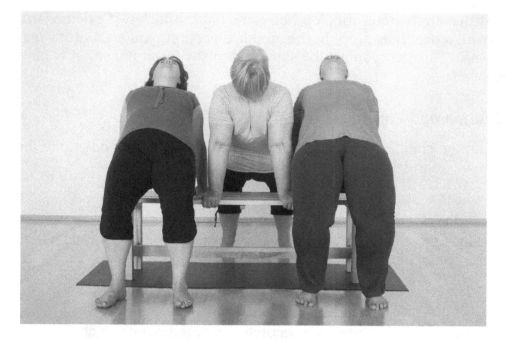

■ Exhaling, move back into the starting position.
■ Repeat the movement during six full inhalations and exhalations.
■ Again, come into the table posture and keep it for three complete inhalations and exhalations.
■ Finally, get back into the seated posture and relax. Feel the space between your shoulder blades. Close your eyes if it feels comfortable for you.

Seated Postures and Rotations

Rotations straighten the spine and help correct crooked postures (scoliosis). Rotations of the extremities mobilize the joints and strengthen the muscles that lead the action or hold the posture during a pause. It is vital to inhale and stretch the vertebrae before you exhale and rotate.

Rotations allow you to feel the polarity of your body. For example, it may be easier for you to turn to one side than to the other. This is often the case. These differences can diminish while you practice yoga. Therefore, it is important to pause after exercising to one side; return to the starting position and feel the difference between both sides. If you continue the exercise on the other side and compare the reaction in both sides of your body again, you will feel more adjusted. This feeling of balance and stability is very relaxing. Rotations are ideal postures in any antistress program.

HEAD ROTATION

Purposes

The head rotation mobilizes your cervical joints and enhances the flexibility of your neck and shoulder muscles. It should be among your daily yoga exercises.

Notes of Caution and Contraindications

If you suffer from a painful neck and soreness in your shoulders, start with moderate movements. Warmth can often support the joint mobility (i.e., from a heating pad or hot water bottle). Although we can turn and bow our head at the same time, it is better to do these joint movements separately or do them in succession. This way, we become aware of the different head movements and exercise safely.

Alignments

To maximize the rotation of your spine, it is necessary to stretch the complete spinal column and create space for the vertebrae and discs. Rotations of the spine should always start with an inhalation and profound stretch. Start with small rotations and expand them through regular practice.

What to Do

- Come into upright seated posture on a chair.
- Your pelvis is in an upright position, your spine is stretched, and your chin is parallel to the floor. Your shoulders and arms are relaxed, along with your face and tongue muscles.
- Place your hands on top of your thighs.
- As you inhale, stretch your spinal column and your neck.
- Exhaling, relax your shoulders.

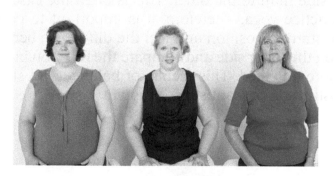

■ Inhaling, turn your head to the right. Make sure that your chin is parallel to the floor, that your head does not bow, and that your shoulders stay relaxed.

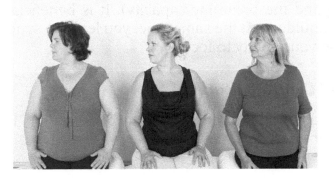

■ Exhaling, turn your head to the left without bowing.

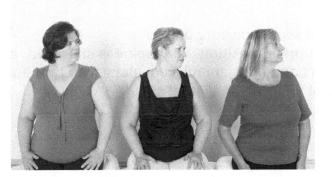

■ Repeat the rotations for six complete inhalations and exhalations.
■ Get back into your initial posture. Feel the effect of the rotations. You may close your eyes if you like.

HEAD AND ARM COORDINATION

Purposes

This coordinating movement helps you relieve tensions in your neck and shoulders and widen your chest (expand the breathing capacity). It is beneficial to prevent headaches that stem from tense shoulders. At the same time, you learn to synchronize movement and breathing and increase your ability to focus.

Notes of Caution and Contraindications

The head and arm coordination is a very gentle way of exercising. It is one of the best ways to perform head rotations and head bows.

Alignments

Make sure that you keep your spine in a stretched and upright position whether you are sitting on your mat or on a chair. Focus on your hand and precisely follow its movements.

What to Do

- Come into an upright seated posture on a chair.
- Your pelvis is in an upright position, your spine is stretched, and your chin is parallel to the floor. Shoulders and arms are relaxed, along with face and tongue muscles. Place your hands on top of your thighs.
- Look down to your right hand.

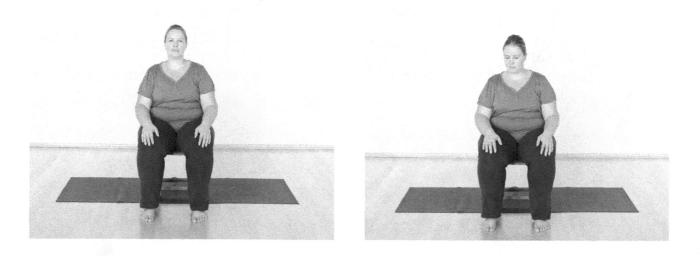

- Inhaling, move your right hand to the right side at shoulder height, and follow the movement with your eyes.
- Look into your right palm as you would look into a mirror.

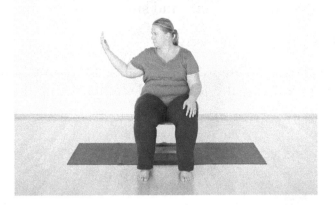

- Exhaling, move your right hand to your left shoulder, and follow the movement with your eyes.

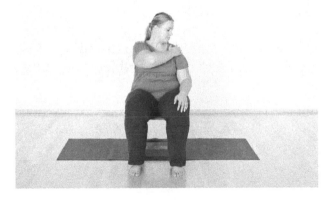

- Inhaling, move your right arm again to the right side, and follow the movement with your eyes. Again look into your palm as you would look into a mirror.
- Exhaling, move your right hand back to your right thigh.
- Continue the exercise: inhaling, move your left hand to the left side, then to your right shoulder, back to the left side, and down to your left thigh.
- Repeat the exercise six times.
- Finally, return to the starting posture and feel the effects in your arms and shoulders. Keep your eyes closed if it feels comfortable.

ARM ROTATION WITH OUTSTRETCHED ARMS

Purposes

Arm rotations can counter a tight chest and a round upper back. At the same time, the rotations mobilize the shoulder and arm joints and strengthen the supporting muscles.

Notes of Caution and Contraindications

Do not be over eager or move too vigorously. Rotations are only helpful if they are carried out in a controlled way, mobilizing the joints and strengthening the supporting muscles.

Alignments

Keep your arms fully stretched and at shoulder height. Exercise with your spine in an upright position.

What to Do

- Come into upright seated posture on a chair.
- Your pelvis is in an upright position, your spine is stretched, and your chin is parallel to the floor. Shoulders and arms are relaxed, along with face and tongue muscles.
- Place your hands on top of your thighs.
- Inhaling through your nose, slowly raise your arms sideways to shoulder height with your palms facing the floor. Make sure that you do not arch your shoulders. If you are not exactly sure, arch your shoulders briefly and let them sink again.

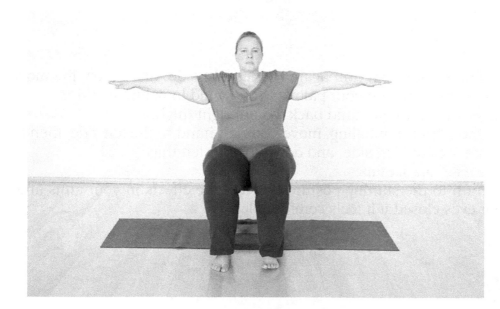

- Exhaling through your nose, rotate your stretched arm backward until your palms face the ceiling.
- Inhaling, rotate your stretched arm forward until your palms face the ceiling again.

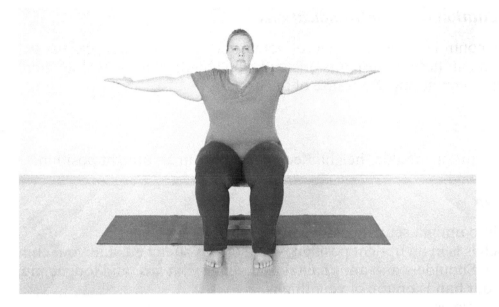

- Repeat this rotation of your stretched arms six times.
- With an exhalation, slowly lower your arms.
- Rest your arms on your thighs and feel the effects. Close your eyes if it feels comfortable.

ARM ROTATION WITH BENT ARMS

Purposes

With this exercise, you rotate your bent arms and feel the difference between pulling your shoulders backward and forward. While rotating your bent arms, you stretch your chest muscles.

Notes of Caution and Contraindications

It is vital to control the movement if you rotate your extremities. If you just swing your arms around, you can harm your joints. Instead, you should start with slow, small movements and expand them during the course of the exercise.

Alignments

Keep your arms at shoulder height. Keep your spine in an upright position.

What to Do

- Come into upright seated posture on a chair.
- Your pelvis is in an upright position, your spine is stretched, and your chin is parallel to the floor. Shoulders and arms are relaxed, along with face and tongue muscles.
- Place your hands on top of your thighs.
- Inhaling, slowly raise your arms sideways to shoulder height. Make sure that you are raising your arms only, not your shoulders. If you are uncertain, briefly arch your shoulders and let them sink again.

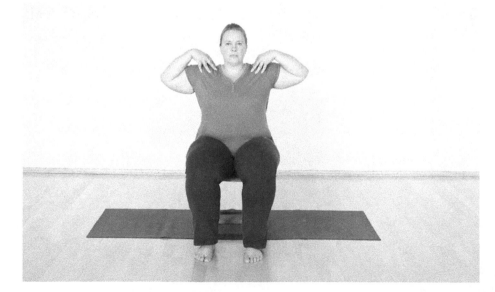

- Exhaling, bend both arms up so that your hands touch the tops of your shoulders.
- Gently rotate your shoulders forward starting with small circles and enlarging them during the course of the exercise.

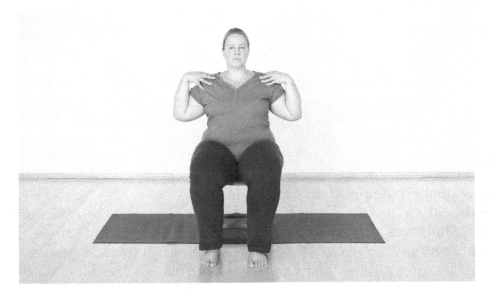

- Keep a steady breathing rhythm that matches the rotations.
- Continue the gentle movement in a forward rotation for at least six inhalations and exhalations.
- Change the direction and gently rotate backward for at least six inhalations and exhalations.
- You can do the exercise with your eyes closed.
- Exhaling, lower your arms. Rest your hands on your thighs, and feel the effects in your shoulders and arms.

HAND LOTUS POSTURE

Purposes

These gentle rotations will ease stiff, painful fingers and wrists.

Notes of Caution and Contraindications

There are no contraindications if you practice thoughtfully, gently mobilizing the joints.

Alignments

Make sure that your wrists are closely connected during the complete movement. Keep your elbows at shoulder height and your spine in an upright position.

What to Do

- Come into upright seated posture on a chair.
- Your pelvis is in an upright position, your spine is stretched, and your chin is parallel to the floor. Shoulders and arms are relaxed, along with face and tongue muscles.
- Inhaling, lift your arms and elbows to chest height. Push palms together.

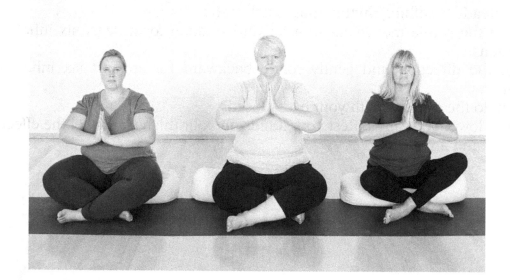

■ Put the tips of both your index fingers and thumbs together to form a nice circle and relax the other fingers.

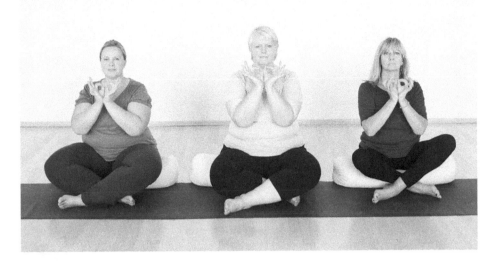

■ Gently rotate your hands and forearms outward. Both wrists are moving around one another until the back of your hands meet with your fingers pointing downward.

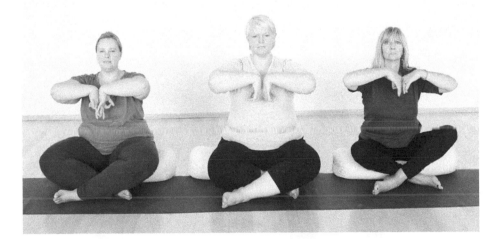

■ Continue the rotation until your fingers point upward again.
■ Remain in a breathing rhythm that matches the gentle rotations.
■ Continue the gentle movement for six inhalations and exhalations.
■ Change the direction, and gently rotate your hands and forearms inward for another six inhalations and exhalations.
■ You can do the exercise with your eyes closed.
■ Exhaling, lower your arms into your lap and feel the effects in your wrists.

Kneeling Postures

If kneeling on your heels or lower legs is difficult on your knees, try the variations demonstrated in this chapter. Make use of a bolster (such as a folded blanket) and place it under either your knees or your feet. It is vital to find a comfortable kneeling posture that you can maintain for a while.

SITTING ON THE HEELS

Purposes

Sitting on the heels mobilizes the knee joints and supports an upright seated posture. You need a bit of practice in order to be able to enjoy this calming and supportive posture for concentration and meditation. It is also a very beneficial posture for numerous breathing techniques and can function as a starting position.

Notes of Caution and Contraindications

People with knee problems should consult their doctor. All others can gently start practicing kneeling postures. Steady and gentle practice will reward you with pain-free knee movements while walking, climbing stairs, riding a bike, dancing, sitting, and standing.

Alignments

Your knees and ankles should not hurt from being in a kneeling posture: Use bolsters. Your heels are not tipped inward or outward. The spinal column is stretched out from your sit bones to the crown of your head.

What to Do

- Kneel on your mat with your feet stretched out. Lower your bottom until your sit bones meet with your heels. Make sure that your heels are not tipped inward or outward. Your knees are a hip width apart.
- Your pelvis is upright, your bottom (or better, your pelvic muscles) are tight, and your belly is relaxed.
- Your spinal column is straightened, and your sternum is raised.
- Your shoulders and arms are relaxed, and your hands are resting on your thighs.
- Your chin is parallel to the floor.
- Your face and mouth muscles are relaxed.
- Completely breathe in and out through your nose.

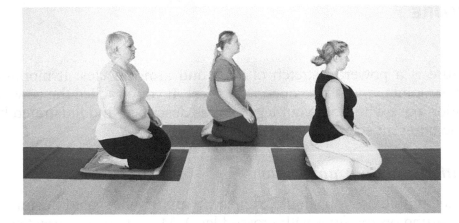

Variation with a Blanket under Knees and Shins

The position of the prop helps you to relieve pressure on your knees and shins.

■ Place a folded blanket under your knees and ankles and recognize the effect.

Variation with a Blanket or Cushion under the Ankles

A folded blanket under your ankles is helpful if your insteps hurt in the kneeling posture.

■ Place a rolled-up blanket or cushion under your insteps and recognize the effect.

Variation with a Cushion between Thighs and Calves

In case you cannot comfortably sit on your heels, a bolster between your thighs and calves allows you a longer and more comfortable rest in the kneeling posture.

■ Place a cushion between your thighs and calves and recognize the effect. Compare the effects and choose the right prop and position for you.

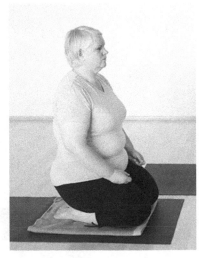
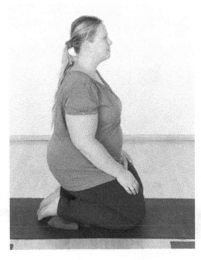
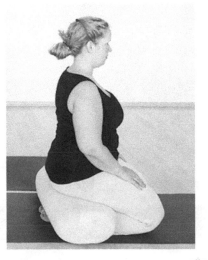

COW POSTURE

Purposes

The cow posture is a powerful stretch of back and arm muscles. It mobilizes shoulder, elbow, and finger joints, and it also opens the chest. If you practice the cow posture in the hero's meditation pose with both your legs bent as described and illustrated here, you will also stretch the outer muscles of the thighs.

Notes of Caution and Contraindications

If you have knee problems, you should exercise in an upright seated posture on a chair or in a free seat (sitting on the floor with crossed legs). Make sure you practice thoughtfully, gently stretching your arm muscles and smoothly mobilizing the joints. Use props instead of forcefully bringing your hands together.

Alignments

Make sure your spine is stretched out and in an upright position. Do not bow forward. Use a prop if necessary.

What to Do

- Come into seated posture on the mat.
- Your pelvis is in an upright position, your spine is stretched, and your chin is parallel to the floor. Your shoulders and arms are relaxed, along with your face and tongue muscles.
- Bend your left leg and place your left foot at the outer side of your right hip. Bend your right leg and place your right foot at the outer side of your left hip. Make sure that both knees are in line. Sit on a bolster if it feels more comfortable.
- With an inhalation, lift both arms. Relax your shoulder muscles.

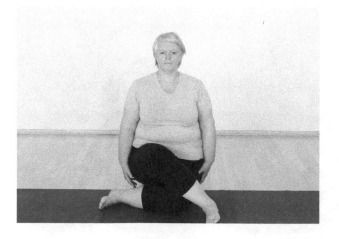 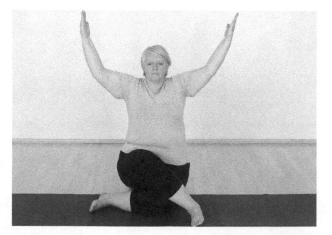

- Bend your left arm and use your right hand to gently pull your left elbow toward the middle of your back.
- With another inhalation, stretch your spine.
- Keep the stretched-out position, and move your right arm behind your torso.
- Move your right arm upward until both your hands meet. Use a strap or towel in the beginning and do not force your hands together. Enjoy a gentle and steady practice.
- Turn your head and look upward to your left elbow.

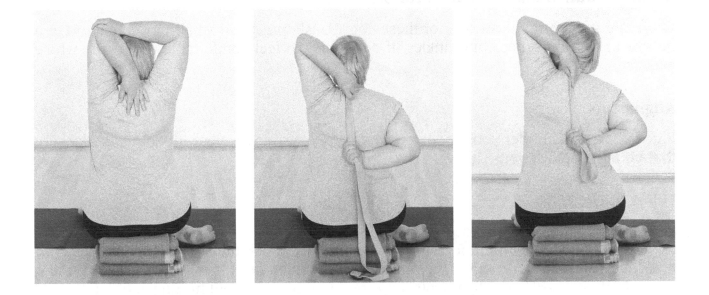

- Keep the posture for six complete inhalations and exhalations.
- With an exhalation, bring your arms back into starting position, and place your hands on top of your upper knee. Compare the feeling in both sides of your body, both sides of your face and shoulder, and in both of your arms.
- Change the position of your legs, and repeat the posture to the other side with your left arm up.
- Finally, come into the seated posture and feel the effect of the whole asana. Close your eyes if it feels comfortable.

TIGER POSTURE

Purposes

The tiger posture mobilizes your spine from the base (sacrum and coccyx) to the top (cervical vertebrae). Your breath leads the movement of the vertebrae. You consciously stretch and bow your spine to become aware of how your back feels in different positions.

Notes of Caution and Contraindications

There are no contraindications for these consciously practiced small movements. Use a bolster under your knees and ankles (if necessary) to feel comfortable during the whole exercise.

Alignments

Place your wrists under your shoulders and your knees under your hip joints. Make sure that you do not lock your elbows.

What to Do

- Come into the kneeling posture.
- With an inhalation, bend forward until your hands touch the floor.
- Make sure that your wrists are under your shoulders and that your knees are under your hip joints. These alignments help you to exercise without hurting your joints.

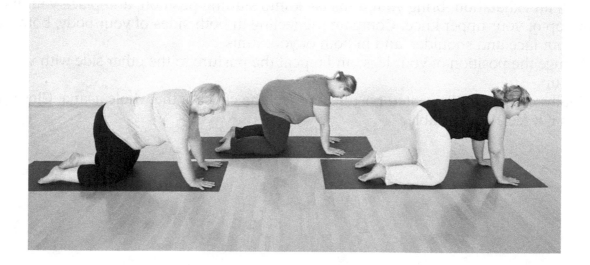

■ On the exhalation, bend your spine vertebra by vertebra. Start at your tailbone and move all the way up: lumbar, thoracic, to cervical spine. Bow your head at the end of the movement.

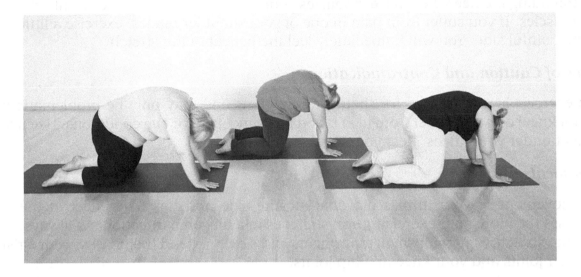

■ On the inhalation, stretch your spine vertebra by vertebra. Start at your tailbone and move all the way up: lumbar, thoracic, to cervical spine. Lift your head at the end of the movement.

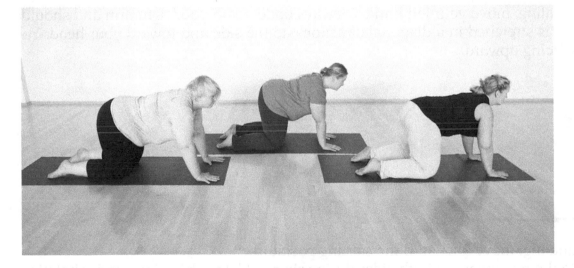

■ Synchronize breathing and moving, and repeat the exercise during six complete inhalations and exhalations.
■ Inhaling, return to the kneeling posture. Place your fingers on top of your thighs and relax. Feel the effects with your eyes closed if it is comfortable.

THREADING THE NEEDLE POSTURE

Purposes

The threading the needle exercise mobilizes your shoulders and stretches trunk, chest, and arm muscles. If you suffer from pain in one of your shoulder blades, exercise a little longer on the painful side. You will immediately feel the benefit of the stretch.

Notes of Caution and Contraindications

This exercise is very helpful for shoulder conditions and may only be problematic if you cannot kneel or if you suffer from high blood pressure or ear or eye conditions. Use a folded blanket under your knees. Rest your head on a bolster.

Alignments

The movement of your arm is diagonal—to the side and top. The effect of the asana increases the more your exercising arm stretches in a diagonal direction. As always, do not force the stretch. Start with small movements and slowly extend them. Align your wrist and shoulder joints and your knee and hip joints.

What to Do

- Start from the kneeling posture and get into the tiger posture (on all fours).
- Make sure that your wrists are underneath your shoulders and that your knees are underneath your hip joints. These alignments help you to exercise without hurting your joints.
- Exhaling, move your left hand sideways underneath your right arm and shoulder. Your arm is stretched in a diagonal direction—to the side and toward your head. Your palm is facing upward.

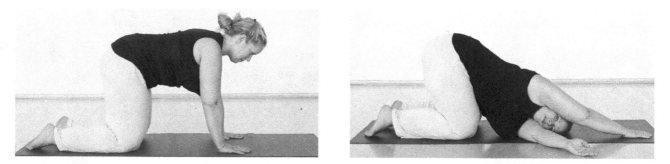

- Inhaling, move back into the starting position.
- Do the movement to both sides during six complete exhalations and inhalations.
- With the next exhalation keep the position, rest your head on one side, and stretch out your upper arm. Keep the asana for six complete inhalations and exhalations.
- Inhaling, get back into the starting position. Compare both sides.
- Do the asana on the other side.
- Finally, get back into the kneeling posture, and place your fingers on top of your thighs. Feel the effects with your eyes closed if you like.

TORSO ROTATION

Purposes

The torso rotation is one of several exercises that mobilize the joints of the thoracic verte-brae. In daily life, we mostly rotate our complete torso at waist height, or we completely turn around if rotating the spine feels difficult. Therefore, it is an uncommon and fairly large stretch for beginners. At the same time, it is not a difficult asana. Next time you sit in a car and turn around you will notice the benefit of this asana—or remember to do the exercise again.

Notes of Caution and Contraindications

The asana cannot be recommended to those who suffer from high blood pressure or ear or eye conditions. If it is difficult for you to kneel, take a cushion or bolster to make the posture more comfortable for you.

Alignments

Keep the exercising arm in a bent position and follow the movement with your eyes to fully rotate your upper spine. Align your elbows and shoulder joints and your knees and hip joints.

What to Do

■ Start from the kneeling posture and get into the tiger posture (on all fours).
■ Exhale and place your forearms on the floor. Your right forearm is in front.

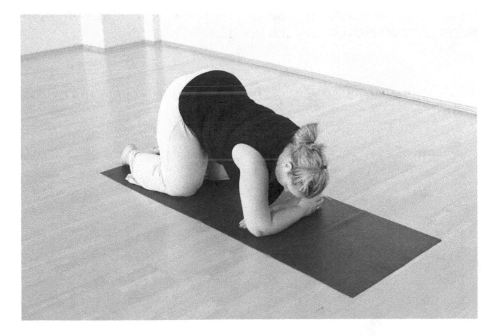

- Make sure that your elbows are underneath your shoulders and that your knees are underneath your hip joints. These alignments help you to exercise without hurting your joints.
- Inhaling, rotate your upper torso, and move your right elbow upward. Make sure that you keep your upper arm bent.

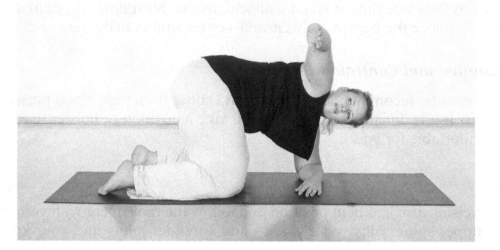

- Exhaling, move back into the starting position.
- Inhaling, rotate your upper torso, and move your left elbow upward. Make sure that you keep your upper arm bent.
- Exhaling, move back into the starting position.
- Repeat the movement to both sides during six complete exhalations and inhalations.
- Finally, get back into the kneeling posture, and place your hands on top of your thighs. Feel the effects with your eyes closed if you like.

CHILD POSTURE

Purposes

In the child posture, you stretch your arm and back muscles. It can also be a comfortable posture in which to rest and feel the effects of your exercises. To fully enjoy this very calming and relaxing asana, you can use bolsters. If you are a beginner or if you want to do this exercise during the day, you can enjoy the stretch in the child posture using two chairs (see the variation later in this section).

Notes of Caution and Contraindications

Become aware which variation works best for you to get a good stretch and a safe and gentle mobilization of your joints. Keep your head above heart level if necessary.

Alignments

Completely stretch your arms and spine. Do not rotate your heels. Depending on your special needs, use bolsters. Make sure that you can comfortably rest on your heels or cushion. Place your head with your forehead on the floor or cushion, and stay at ease.

What to Do

- Start from the kneeling posture and get into the tiger posture (on all fours).
- Make sure that your wrists are underneath your shoulders and that your knees are underneath your hip joints. These alignments help you to exercise without hurting your joints.
- Exhaling, bend your knees and lower your chest until your bottom meets with your heels (or cushion).
- Stretch out your arms and place your palms shoulder width apart on the floor.

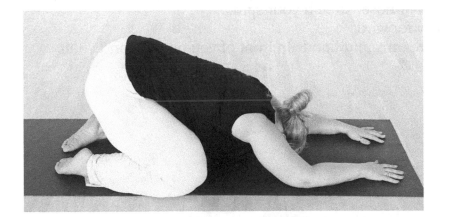

- Keep the posture for six complete inhalations and exhalations.
- Inhaling, move into the tiger posture.
- With another inhalation, roll up into the kneeling posture.
- Place your hands on your thighs, and feel the effects with your eyes closed if you would like to do so.

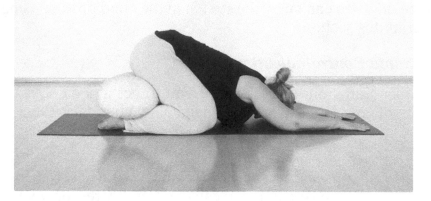

Variation with a Bolster

If you want to keep the position for a while, try a bolster.

- Place a bolster between your thighs and your lower legs.

Variation with Two Chairs

During the day you can stretch your back and arm muscles in an easy way. Use two chairs.

- Start in an upright seated posture on a chair.
- Place your feet more than hip width apart and rest your hands in your lap. While inhaling through your nose, stretch your spine.
- Exhaling, bow forward.
- Place your forearms and hands in front of you on a second chair.

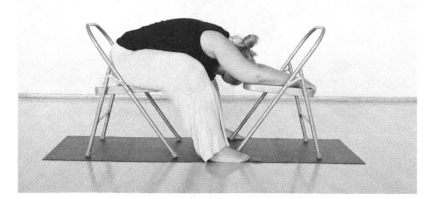

CHILD AND TIGER POSTURE

The combination of tiger and child posture allows your spine to smoothly and continuously bow backward and forward in a safe posture on your mat. It might be helpful if you think of a wave to get into the flowing motion of the child-tiger-child-asana. See the detailed description of both asanas earlier.

What to Do

- Come into the tiger posture (kneeling on all fours). Make sure that your wrists are underneath your shoulders and your knees are underneath your hip joints. These alignments help you to exercise without hurting your joints.
- Exhaling, move backward into the child posture.
- Lower your chin toward your chest.
- Inhaling, raise into the tiger posture and stretch your spine vertebra by vertebra. Start this stretch at the bottom (sacrum and coccyx) and proceed with each vertebra of your lumbar (lower back), thoracic (middle), and cervical (closest to your skull) spine. Finally, raise your head. At the end of the inhalation, your spine is fully stretched and you are looking downward to the floor.

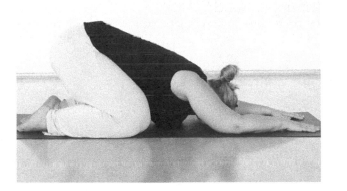 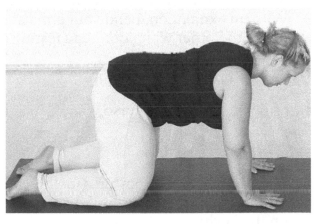

- Exhaling, move backward until your buttocks touches your heels (or cushion). Slowly bend your spine vertebra by vertebra. Start at the bottom and end with a head bow. Feel your chin meeting with your chest.
- Inhaling, move into tiger posture, and continue the asana in a constant flow.
- Continue in the flowing motion for at least six complete inhalations and exhalations. Synchronize breathing and moving and enjoy the flow.
- Finally, get back into the starting posture and rise into the kneeling posture. Place your hands on your thighs and feel the effects with your eyes closed if you like.

MODIFIED FOLDED LEAF POSTURE

In the folded leaf posture, you rest your forehead on your mat and your arms alongside your lower legs with your palms facing the ceiling. As opposed to the child posture, the modified folded leaf posture does not stretch the arm muscles. This posture is beneficial if you completely rest your arms and relax your shoulders. It feels more comfortable for a beginner if you try the modified version or use a bolster. With each exhalation, further lower your shoulders toward the mat or cushion, and with each inhalation feel the bow of your spine.

Notes of Caution and Contraindications

There are no contraindications for the modified folded leaf posture. Keep your head above heart level if necessary.

Alignments

Completely relax your arms and shoulders.

What to Do

- Start from the child posture (for the variation with a cushion, see earlier).
- With an exhalation, bend your arms and place your hands in front of you, one hand on top of the other with your head resting on your upper hand.

Variation with Two Cushions

To completely rest your torso, shoulders, and head, use two bolsters.

What to Do

- Start from the child posture (for the variation with a cushion see earlier).
- Place a second cushion in front of you and fully relax your torso, head, and shoulders on the cushion.

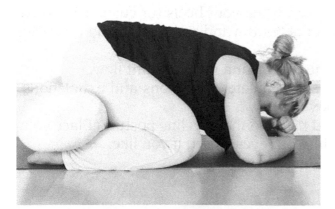 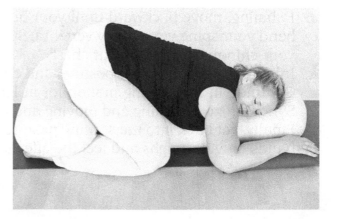

MODIFIED SIDE REST

Purposes

The side rest strengthens your hand, arm, and shoulder muscles and mobilizes your wrist, elbow, and shoulder joints. In this posture, your flanks are stretched, and your sense of balance is challenged. The modified version lessens the strain on the joints. You benefit from the exercise without hurting your joints and risking a fall.

Notes of Caution and Contraindications

There are no contraindications for the modified version of the side rest.

Alignments

Place your wrists under your shoulders, and do not lock your elbows. Completely stretch your back, tighten your pelvic muscles, and keep your arms in a line.

What to Do

- Come into the kneeling posture.
- With an inhalation, bend forward until your hands touch the floor (on all fours).
- Make sure that your wrists are under your shoulders and your knees are under your hip joints.

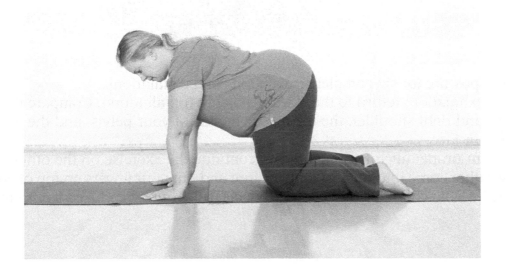

- Spread your hands and place your palms flat on your mat. This position allows for better distribution of the weight that your hand will carry in the side rest.
- On the inhalation, stretch your left leg and place your left foot with its inner side on your mat.
- Use the exhalation to check the stable position of your hands and your left foot.
- On the next inhalation, lift your left arm and rotate your body backward until your arms are in line.
- Use the next exhalation to stretch your back and pelvic muscles and to stabilize the position of your right hand and your left foot.

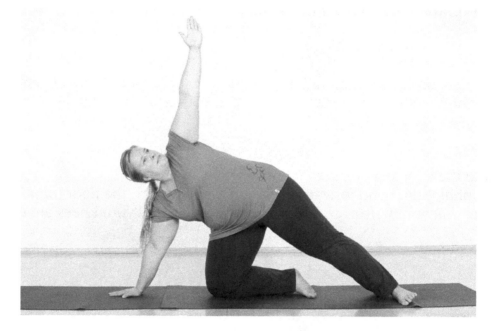

- Keep the posture for six complete inhalations and exhalations.
- With an exhalation, return to the starting posture (on all fours). Compare the feeling in your left and right shoulder, the left and right side of your pelvis, and the left and right side of your face.
- Check your proper alignment before you continue the exercise on the other side.
- Finally, either come into the kneeling posture and put your fingers on top of your thighs, or come into the child posture. Feel the effects with your eyes closed if it is comfortable.

Standing Postures and Bows

Standing postures are done with a stretched spine, often in combination with a bow—forward, sideward, and backward. If you are not sure about the proper alignment of your spine, you can use a wall as a prop. Your heels, bottom, and shoulders should always be in contact with the wall.

UPRIGHT STANDING POSTURE

Purposes

This upright standing posture is also called tadasana or mountain posture. If you learn to do it properly, you can practice it during the day while waiting in line, while waiting for an elevator, or while talking on the phone. You will feel an immediate uplifting effect if you raise yourself up and stand tall. Do not forget to lower your shoulders and relax your face and tongue. After some practice, you will feel the strength of the posture in both body and mind.

Notes of Caution and Contraindications

There are no general contraindications for the upright standing posture.

Alignments

Keep your spine fully stretched out. In profile, your shoulder, hip, knee, and ankle are in line.

What to Do

- Place your feet hip width apart, and distribute the weight of your body evenly on your feet. If you feel more weight on the inner side of your feet (a tendency toward standing knock-kneed), make sure that you correct your weight distribution toward the outer edges of your feet (and vice versa).
- Extend your knees without hyperextending them.
- Rotate your thighs outward, keep your feet in place, and feel your pelvis lifting up.
- Support the position of your pelvis by tightening your pelvic muscles.
- Stretch your vertebrae between your tailbone and the crown of your head.
- Your belly is relaxed.
- Your sternum is raised, and your shoulders and arms hang down loosely.

■ Your chin is parallel to the ground, and your face, lips, and tongue are relaxed.
■ Breathe in and out deeply through your nose.

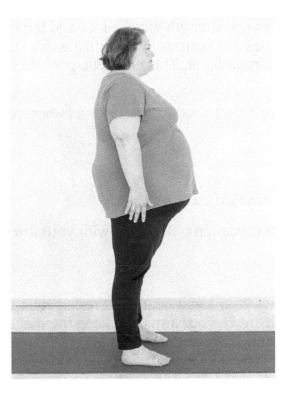

HERO 2 POSTURE

Purposes

The hero 2 posture enhances the strength of your foot and leg muscles. Small adjustments in the feet and spine muscles are constantly stabilizing the stance, and a good sense of balance is necessary for maintaining it. This energetic posture will boost your mood.

"My favorite asana is the hero 2 posture. I feel powerful whenever I am in this posture."
—Anika

Notes of Caution and Contraindications

There are no general contraindications. Be gentle with your knees and stay aligned.

Alignments

Stretch your spine and keep your torso centered. Your pelvis is in line with the ankle of your forward pointing foot. Stretch your arms and keep them at shoulder level. The posture is perfect if your ankles are under your knees.

What to Do

- Come into the upright standing posture.
- Turn your right foot completely outward, and take a step forward in the same direction.
- Turn your left foot 45 degrees inward. Make sure that your pelvis is in the same position it was when you started.

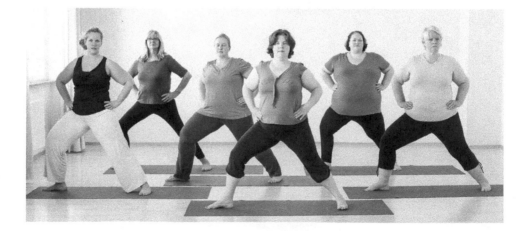

- Inhaling, raise your arms to shoulder height. Stretch out both arms and keep the stretch. Feel the stretch in your arms and in your fingertips.
- Exhaling, slowly bend your right knee forward.
- Turn your head and look along your outstretched right arm. Make sure that your torso is in an upright position; do not bend forward.

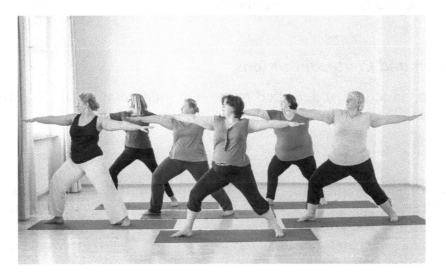

- Keep the position for six full inhalations and exhalations.
- With an inhalation, stretch both legs and lower your arms.
- Bring your feet into the starting position, and compare both sides of your body—both legs, both sides of your pelvis, both shoulders, both sides of your face.
- Repeat the posture with your other foot in front.
- Finally, return to the standing posture, and feel the energy in your body. Close your eyes if you like.

MODIFIED MOUNTAIN POSTURE

Purposes

The modified mountain posture (depending on the yoga tradition, this is also called the downward-facing dog posture) stretches your backside from the heels to the top of your fingers. It enhances the flexibility of the muscles on the back side of your legs, pelvis, and torso.

Notes of Caution and Contraindications

If you suffer from glaucoma, a detached retina, ear inflammation, or high blood pressure, keep your head above heart level. Practice the modified posture and use a chair as prop.

Alignments

Make sure the chair does not slide. Keep your ankles, knees, and hip joints in one line. Your arms are stretched and in line with your stretched spine. Look downward to include your neck in the full spinal stretch.

What to Do

- Come into the upright standing posture.
- Position a chair in front of you. Make sure that the chair cannot slide away.
- Place your hands on your thighs and bend your knees.
- On the exhalation, lower your torso until it is parallel to the floor.
- On the inhalation, stretch your arms and place your hands on the seat of the chair.

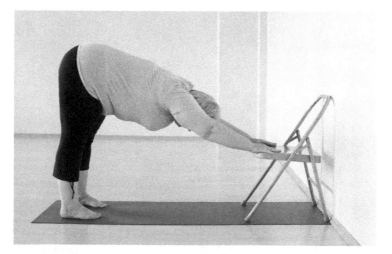

- You can also grasp the seat of the chair if it feels more secure that way.

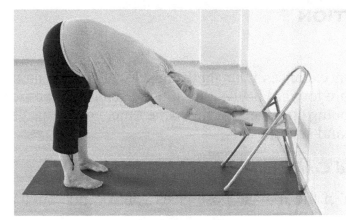

- Stretch out your arms and your back (including your neck), and keep your ankles, knees, and hip joints aligned.
- Stay in the position for six complete inhalations and exhalations.
- On an inhalation, slowly roll up into the standing posture. You can bend your knees if it feels more comfortable.
- Feel the stretch in your arms, back, and legs. Close your eyes if it feels comfortable.

Variation with Head above Heart Level

To keep your head above heart level, use the back of a chair as prop.

What to Do

- Come into the upright standing posture.
- Position a chair in front of you. Make sure that the chair cannot slide away.
- Place your hands on your thighs and bend your knees.
- On the exhalation, lower your torso until it is parallel to the floor.
- On the inhalation, stretch your arms and place your hands on the back of a chair.

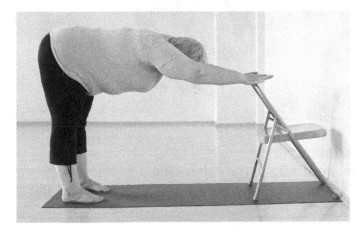

TRIANGLE IN MOTION

Purposes

The triangle in motion exercises your flank muscles. Because most of the bows we are doing during the day are forward bows, it is vital to exercise to the side and stretch a group of muscles that miss being stretched. At the same time, your arms get stretched overhead, and your wrists bend and stretch.

Notes of Caution and Contraindications

This modified version of the triangle pose gives you a gentle stretch and has no general contraindications.

Alignments

It is vital to exercise to the side and stretch the flanks.

What to Do

- Come into the upright standing posture.
- Shift your weight to your right foot.
- With an inhalation:
  - move your left foot in front of your right foot,
  - move your left arm in front of your belly (bend your left hand),
  - lift your right arm (bend your right hand), and
  - turn your head to the left.

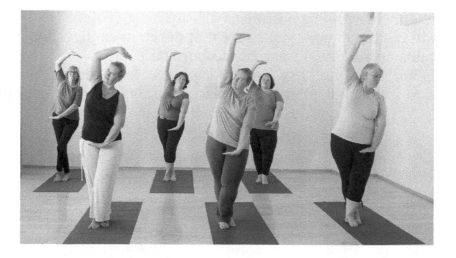

- Pause with an exhalation.
- With an inhalation, continue to the other side.
- Finally, exhaling, return into the starting posture, and feel the effects of the exercise. Close your eyes if it feels comfortable.

HALF MOON POSTURE

Purposes

The half moon posture is a demanding bend to the side that strengthens your leg muscles and challenges your sense of balance. It will be easier if you start doing this posture with a prop: You can use the wall, a chair, or a block. Exercise one side of the body followed by the other. Notice the differences in each side.

Notes of Caution and Contraindications

If you easily feel dizzy or if you suffer from high blood pressure or eye or ear conditions, do not undertake the full posture.

> "Yoga makes you more flexible; you develop more stamina. I love back bows as well as the half moon posture."
>
> —Denise

Alignments

As a beginner, you should exercise with your back against a wall. Make sure that you start from a secure basic stance.

What to Do

- Come into the upright standing posture.
- Position your feet one length of a leg apart. Turn the right foot outward with the toes pointing forward. Turn the left foot inward.
- While breathing in through your nose, slowly lift your arms over the sides until they are fully stretched out at shoulder height. Make sure that you do not pull up your shoulders. If you are not exactly sure, you can raise your shoulders briefly and let them sink again.
- While exhaling, bend your right knee and place the fingertips of your right hand in front of your right foot on a block (or on a chair). Your left arm is relaxed, and your left hand is on top of your pelvis.
- Inhaling, stretch your right leg and lift your left leg and left arm. The proper alignment is: the left leg is parallel to the floor, and the left arm is in line with the right arm. Your neck is stretched with your head in a balanced position looking forward.

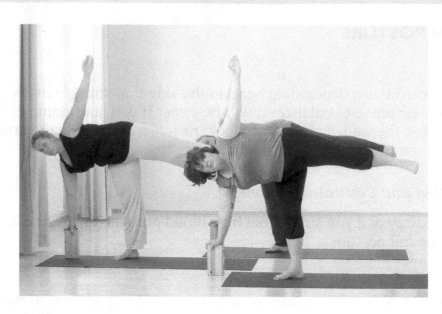

- Keep the posture for six complete inhalations and exhalations.
- To get out of the posture: Inhaling, lift your right arm and your torso, and lower your left leg and left arm.
- Come into the standing posture, and compare the feeling in both sides of your body—your legs, both sides of your pelvis, both shoulders, and both sides of your face. You may close your eyes if you like to do so.
- Repeat the posture to the other side.
- Finally, return to the standing posture, compare both sides again, and feel the effects of the whole balancing exercise. Close your eyes if it is comfortable for you.

HERO I POSTURE

Purposes

In the hero 1 posture, the front of your body is fully stretched in a smooth backbend. With your arms stretched out above your head, the posture works your body from head to toe. The posture strengthens your foot, leg, arm, and shoulder muscles, stretches your complete spine, and mobilizes your shoulder joints. Breathing and moving steadily and rhythmically, you will deepen your breath, increasing the oxygen level of your blood and improving your ability to concentrate.

Notes of Caution and Contraindications

This posture provides a gentle backbend. There are no general contraindications for the hero 1 posture.

Alignments

Keep your feet hip joint width apart. Align your bent knee with your ankle. Stretch your complete spine and keep your pelvic muscles tightened.

What to Do

- Come into the upright standing posture.
- Move your left foot forward. Make sure that your feet are still hip width apart. Keep both legs stretched and both heels on the floor.
- Bring both palms together in front of your sternum.

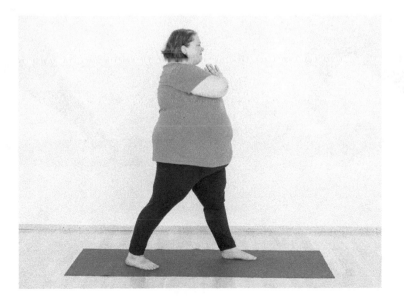

- With an inhalation, slowly lower your front leg, push your elbows backward, and stretch your shoulders. Make sure that you do not lift your shoulders. Keep your front knee properly aligned over your ankle.
- With an exhalation, slowly move back into the starting position with palms together and both knees stretched.
- Repeat the exercise for six full inhalations and exhalations.

If you have a good sense of balance, continue with the asana.

- Inhaling, bend your front knee, stretch out your arms, and look upward.
- Hold this posture for six full inhalations and exhalations.
- Exhaling, return to the starting position.
- Move your front foot backward and return to the standing posture.
- Close your eyes and compare both sides—both legs, both sides of your pelvis, both sides of your face.
- Repeat the exercise with your other foot in front.
- Finally, return to the standing posture, close your eyes, and feel the stretch of your back and the balancing effect of the whole exercise.

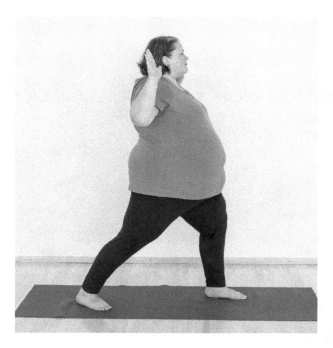 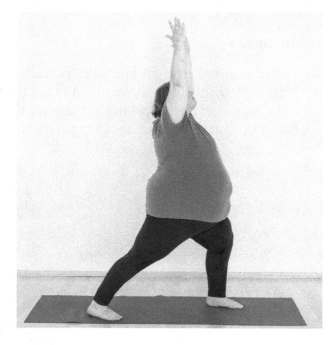

STARGAZER

Purposes

The stargazer posture stretches the chest muscles and mobilizes the shoulder joints. At the same time, it strengthens the feet and leg muscles and develops a sense of balance. While working with our hands, we often bend our neck and shoulders forward and tighten the chest. Unless we work against this poor posture regularly, it can lead to a rounded or humped upper spine.

Notes of Caution and Contraindications

The stargazer is a posture that gently stretches the spine in a backbend and has no contraindications. Instead of looking upward, look ahead if you feel unstable. Cross your arms behind your back if it is difficult for you to bring your hands together behind your back.

Alignments

Both legs are stretched out. Both heels touch the mat. Stretch your complete spine and keep your pelvic muscles tightened.

What to Do

- Come into the upright standing posture.
- Put one foot forward.

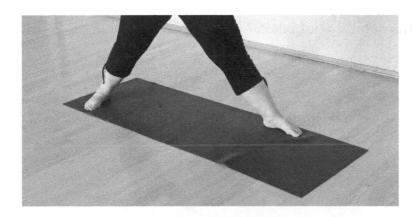

- Make sure that your feet are still hip width apart and that the outer sides of your feet are parallel. Keep both legs stretched and both heels on the floor.
- Bring both palms together behind your back.

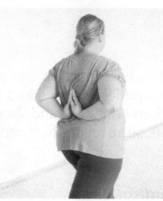

- With an inhalation, stretch your spinal column, bend backward, and look upward. Make sure that your pelvic muscles are tight.
- Keep the position for six full inhalations and exhalations.
- With an inhalation, return to the starting position.
- Move your front foot backward, and get into the standing posture.
- Close your eyes and compare both sides—both legs, both sides of your pelvis, both sides of your face.
- Repeat the exercise with your other foot in front.
- Finally, return to the standing posture, close your eyes, and feel the effect of the whole exercise.

Variation with Your Arms Crossed behind Your Back

If you do not yet have the flexibility to bring your hands together behind your back, try the following variation.

- Cross your arms behind your back.

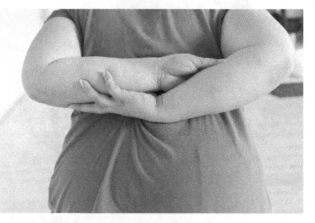

- Notice: When you exercise to the other side (i.e., you started with your left foot in front and will repeat the asana with your right foot in front), change the position of your arms as well. If you had your left arm on top (as in the photo), put your right arm on top while repeating the asana.

STANDING BOW POSTURE

Purposes

The standing bow posture requires a good sense of balance. It provides a noticeable stretch of chest and thigh muscles, mobilizes the shoulder and hip joints, and strengthens the feet and leg muscles. Here, we demonstrate the bow posture with a strap.

Notes of Caution and Contraindications

If you feel unstable and cannot properly bow your leg backward while standing on one foot, take hold of your foot with one hand and touch a wall.

Alignments

Your bent leg has to be parallel to the other leg. Completely stretch your spine before bending backward.

What to Do

- Come into the upright standing posture.
- Tighten your pelvic muscles. Shift your weight to the left foot and leg. Bend your right knee, move both arms backward, and get hold of your right foot with the help of a strap.
- With an inhalation through your nose, stretch your spine in this position.
- With an exhalation through your nose, bend your right thigh backward.
- Make sure that your right leg is not rotating to the side.

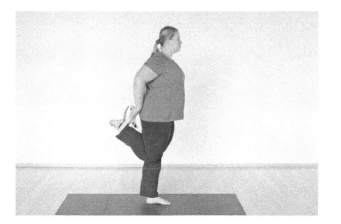

- Keep the posture for six complete inhalations and exhalations.
- With an exhalation, release your knee, stretch your right foot, and place it on the mat.
- Compare both sides of your body—your legs, both sides of your pelvis, your shoulders, and both sides of your face.
- Repeat the posture standing on the other foot.
- Finally, return to the starting position. Feel the effects of the backbend in the standing posture. Close your eyes if it is comfortable for you.

10

Standing Postures with Rotations

Standing postures with rotations mobilize different parts of the spine. To benefit fully from the rotation, it is necessary to stretch the spine first. Keep the following in mind: Inhale, stretch your spine, exhale, and rotate your spine.

TORSO ROTATION

Purposes

The torso rotation is a standing posture that mobilizes the joints of the cervical and thoracic spine and those of your shoulders and arms. If you stand tall with your feet grounded on your mat, it also mobilizes the joints of your feet, legs, and hips. As it only requires a little bit of space and time to practice, this posture is easy to perform throughout your day.

Notes of Caution and Contraindications

There are no general contraindications for the torso rotation.

Alignments

Your arms are at shoulder height during the whole exercise. Your feet are parallel and your soles have full contact with the mat.

What to Do

- Come into the upright standing posture.
- Place your feet more than hip width apart. Make sure both soles and both outer sides of your feet are touching the mat.

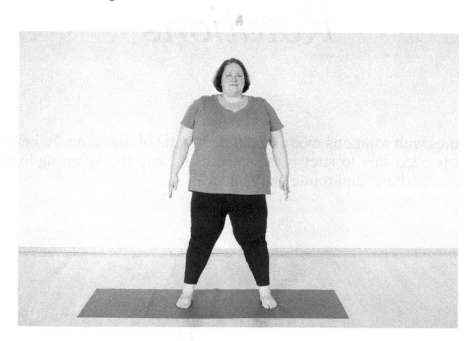

■ Breathe in through your nose, and slowly raise both your arms to shoulder height. Raise your arms, but do not pull up your shoulders. If you are not exactly sure, you can pull up your shoulders briefly and let them sink again.

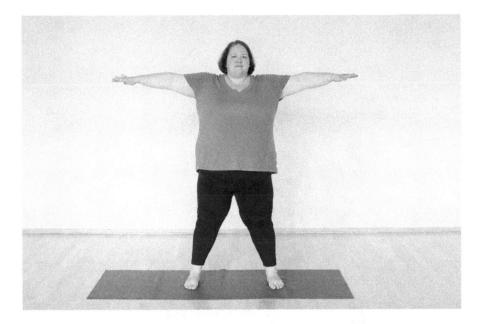

■ Bend your left arm until your hand is in front of your sternum.

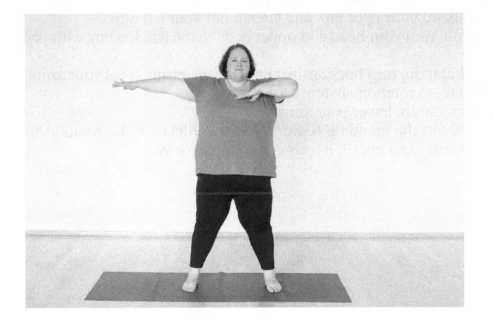

■ Exhaling, turn your outstretched right arm backward and rotate your upper torso and your head to the right. Your right arm is leading the movement.

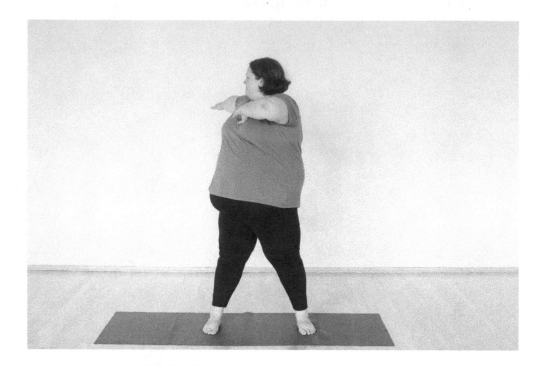

■ With an inhalation, rotate back into the starting posture, and change the position of your arms; bend your right arm and stretch out your left arm.
■ Breathing out, turn your head and upper body to the left, leading with your outstretched left arm.
■ With an inhalation, turn back again, changing the positions of your arms, and continue.
■ Repeat this torso rotation six times.
■ With an exhalation, lower your arms.
■ Finally, while in the standing posture, feel the effects of the rotation in your thoracic vertebrae. Close your eyes if it feels comfortable for you.

HIP ROTATION

Purposes

The hip rotation is a well-known and simple exercise that enhances the mobility of the feet, knee, and hip joints and lifts the mood.

Notes of Caution and Contraindications

There are not contraindications for this exercise.

Alignments

Both feet are firmly on the ground. Slowly extend your movements.

What to Do

- Come into the upright standing posture.
- Put your feet one leg length apart. Make sure both soles and both outer sides of your feet are touching the ground. Extend your knees, making sure not to hyperextend them.
- Place your hands on your hips.

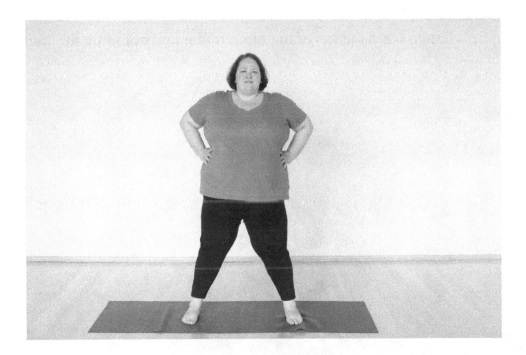

- Slowly start moving your pelvis in a circle and keep to a steady breathing rhythm. Expand the movement.

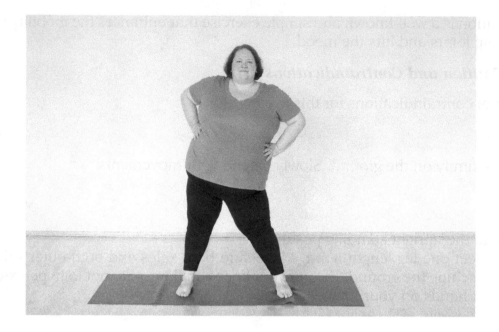

- After a while, change the direction of the hip rotation and continue the exercise.

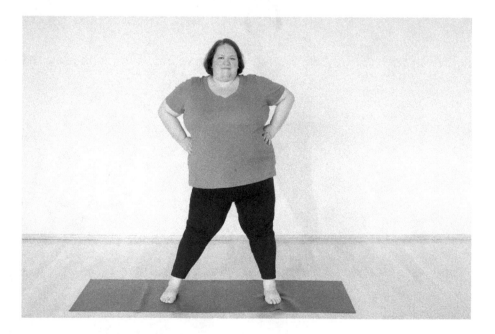

- Finally, stop the rotation and return to the standing posture. Feel the effects of the steady rotation.

KNEE ROTATION

Purposes

Knee rotations in a standing posture can be done almost anywhere. By practicing the knee rotation frequently, you will improve the alignment of your knee joints and help prevent knee problems. This exercise can also be done in a lying posture (see Chapter 3).

Notes of Caution and Contraindications

If you have knee replacements, consult your doctor. It is vital for everybody to exercise with care and control the movements. Start with small rotations and expand them during the course of the exercise.

Alignments

Keep your spine stretched out. Exercise with slow and controlled movements.

What to Do

- Come into the upright standing posture.
- Bend both your knees and put your hands on top of your kneecaps. Your fingers are facing downward.

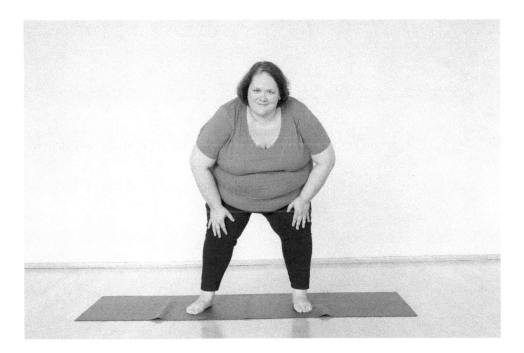

- Fully stretch out your spine, and bow forward with a straight spine.
- Slowly rotate your knees in one direction, and keep to a regular breathing rhythm.
- Continue in the same direction while you do six complete inhalations and exhalations.
- Change the direction, and do the rotation to the opposite side during the next six full breath cycles.
- Gently stop the movement, roll your body upward with your knees bent, come into the standing posture, and feel the effects in your knees. Close your eyes if it feels comfortable for you.

TWISTED TRIANGLE POSTURE

Purposes

The twisted triangle posture exercises your flank muscles, rotates your spine, and enhances your sense of balance. As it is a rather complex exercise, it will also improve your ability to concentrate.

Notes of Caution and Contraindications

This posture needs a bit of yoga practice. If you easily feel unstable or if you suffer from high blood pressure or eye or ear conditions, do not practice the twisted triangle posture.

Alignments

Start from a safe basic stance. Your outstretched arms are in line. You are bending to the side. If your belly gets in the way, use a block.

What to Do

- Come into the upright standing posture.
- Place your feet one leg length apart. Turn your left foot outward with your toes pointing forward. Turn your right foot 45 degrees outward.
- With an inhalation, slowly raise your arms until they are fully stretched out at shoulder height. Make sure that you did not pull up your shoulders. If you are not exactly sure, you can raise your shoulders briefly and let them sink again.
- Exhaling, rotate your torso 180 degrees. Keep your arms stretched out at shoulder level. Inhale and stretch your spine in this position.

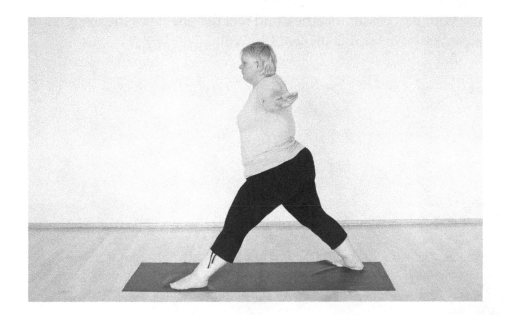

- Exhaling, bend your torso to the side. Your right arm will be moving downward until your fingers can reach the block in front of your left foot. Your left arm is stretched upward toward the ceiling. Make sure that both arms are in line.

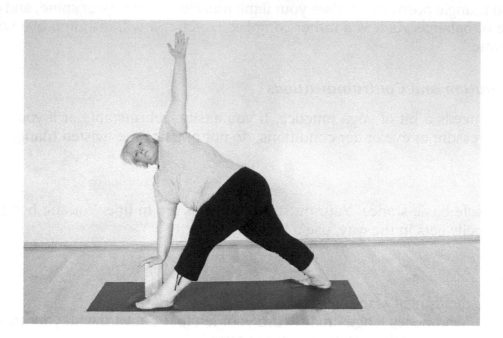

- Keep the twisted triangle posture for six complete inhalations and exhalations.
- To get out of the posture: Inhaling, rotate and lift your torso into the starting position.
- Exhaling, lower your arms.
- Close your eyes if you like, and compare the feeling in both sides of your body—both legs, both sides of your pelvis, both shoulders, and both sides of your face.
- Repeat the posture to the other side.
- Finally, bring your feet closer together, and feel the effects of the exercise in the standing posture. Close your eyes if it is pleasant for you.

11

Balancing Postures

All standing postures require a certain amount of balance, but the postures included in this chapter focus on improving your balance. For all these postures, it is vital to start from a proper basic stance and use a chair or wall as a prop to help steady you if necessary. These balancing postures are demonstrated in motion and as static postures.

PALM TREE POSTURE

Purposes

The palm tree posture is practiced standing on the tips of the toes with arms stretched out. It provides a profound stretch and challenges the sense of balance—although you are standing on both feet. It also strengthens the foot and leg muscles. It is a small but effective exercise for short breaks during the day.

Notes of Caution and Contraindications

This exercise is a standing posture with no contraindications. Just make sure that you either use a prop or practice with both feet on the floor if you feel unstable.

Alignments

Your spinal column is stretched out between pelvis and head crown, including the neck. Your arms are stretched above your head, and your shoulders, your face, and your tongue are relaxed. Your breath flows in and out through the nose.

What to Do

- Come into the upright standing posture.
- Cross your fingers and lay your hands on your head with your palms facing the ceiling.
- Inhaling through your nose, stretch your arms and lift your heels until your weight is balanced on the tips of your toes.
- Exhaling through your nose, lower your arms to your sides, and place your feet back on the mat with the weight evenly spread over your soles.
- Repeat the movement during six complete inhalations and exhalations.
- Finally, return to the standing posture, and feel the energy in your feet and the effects of the balancing posture. If it is comfortable, close your eyes.

Variation with a Prop

If you cannot stay on the tips of your toes during six complete inhalations and exhalations, use a prop.

- Place a folded blanket or a rolled-up mat under your heels.

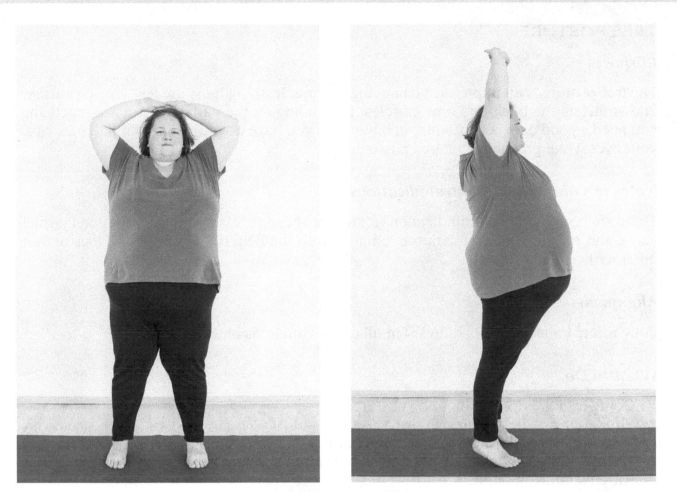

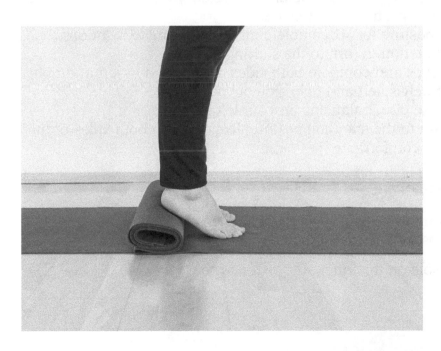

TREE POSTURE

Purposes

The tree posture is an impressive balancing posture. It strengthens the feet and leg muscles and stretches the back and arm muscles. Depending on the variation you are practicing, you need a good or excellent sense of balance. If you have no problems with balance, close your eyes while practicing the tree posture.

Notes of Caution and Contraindications

There are no genuine contraindications for the tree posture. Start with the variation in which you stand on one foot and maintain balance with the help of the tips of the toes of your other foot.

Alignments

Fully rotate your hip joints outward in all of the variations of the tree posture.

What to Do

- Come into the upright standing posture.
- Shift your weight to your right leg.
- Inhaling, bend your left leg—the one not holding your weight—and push the soles of your left foot against the inner side of your inner right ankle. Rotate your bent leg outward as far as possible.
- Fold your fingers. On the inhalation, stretch your arms. Relax your shoulders, face muscles, your lips, and your tongue.
- Stay in this posture for six complete inhalations and exhalations.
- With an exhalation, return to the starting posture.
- Close your eyes and compare both sides of your body—left and right leg, left and right side of your pelvis, left and right side of your face.
- Repeat the exercise, balancing on your left leg.
- Finally, return to the standing posture, feeling again both sides of the body. Close your eyes if it feels comfortable.

Variation on One Foot

If you have enough strength in your feet and legs and a good sense of balance, you can try the following posture.

- Place your sole on the inner side of your knee.

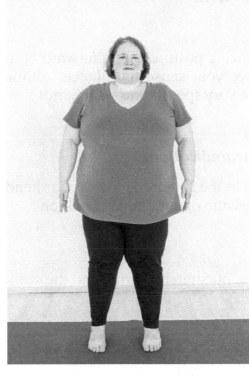

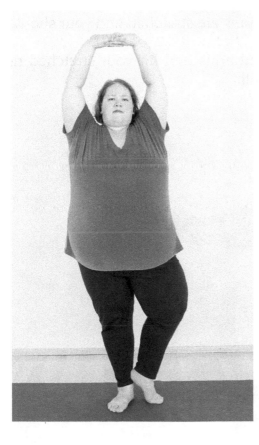

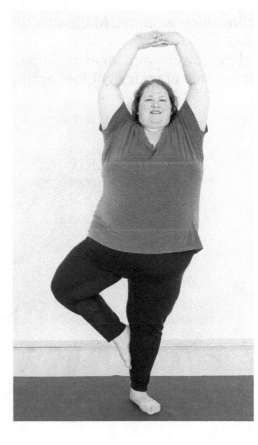

MODIFIED HERO 3 POSTURE

Purposes

The hero 3 posture is a balancing posture with a forward bow. It will strengthen your foot and leg muscles and improve your sense of balance. Although forward bends are very common in daily life, this is a very special one, as it bends the torso while the pelvis pivots around your hip joint.

Notes of Caution and Contraindications

Use a wall or chair as a prop in the beginning. Keep your head above heart level if you are suffering from high blood pressure or ear or eye conditions.

Alignments

The asana is perfect when the outstretched arms and the stretched leg are in line.

What to Do

- Come into the upright standing posture.
- Position your mat in front of a wall.
- Shift your weight to your left leg and foot.
- Inhaling, lift your arms. Make sure that your arms are stretched and your shoulders are relaxed.
- Exhaling, lower your torso and your stretched arms and lift your stretched right leg. Push the sole of your right foot against the wall.

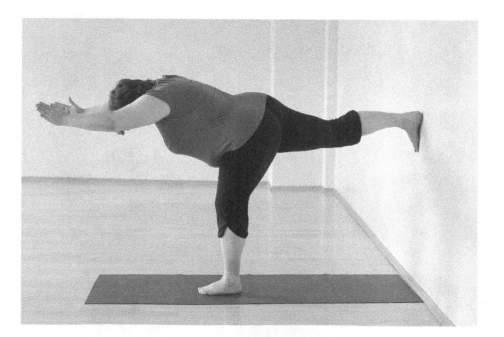

■ Keep the posture for six complete inhalations and exhalations.
■ Inhaling, get back into the starting position. Exhaling, lower your arms to your sides.
■ Close your eyes and compare the feeling in both sides of your body—both legs, both sides of your pelvis, both shoulders, and both sides of your face.
■ Repeat the posture balancing on your right foot.
■ Finally, feel the effects of the exercise in the standing posture. Close your eyes if it is pleasant for you.

Variation with a Chair

If you have trouble keeping the posture—it could be a question of the strength of your feet and legs or of your stability—try the following variation:

■ Position a chair in front of you on your mat.
■ Come into the upright standing posture. Make sure that your arms and shoulders are relaxed.
■ Shift your weight to your left leg and foot.
■ Exhaling, bend your torso downward and your right leg upward. Place your hands on the chair.
■ Keep the posture for six complete inhalations and exhalations.

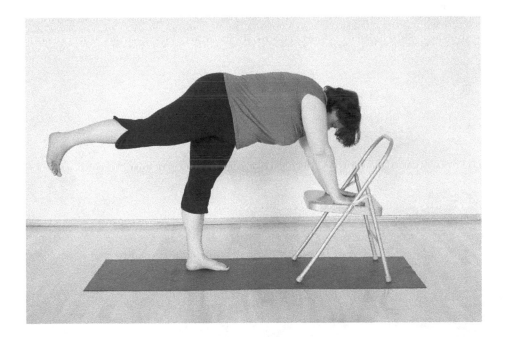

12

Inversions

In all inverted postures, the flow of the blood toward the heart is increased. If you stand on your legs for hours, you will benefit from the inverted postures. If you have high blood pressure or eye or ear conditions do not bow your head below heart level. Use a bolster under your head and try legs up the wall to relieve your legs and feet.

Inversions can put strain on the neck, and some yoga teachers exclude inversions from their classes for bigger people. Here, I have provided modified versions and explain how to use props to perform these postures safely.

"I like the headstand with two chairs as props."
—Céline

MODIFIED SHOULDER STAND

Purposes

The modified shoulder stand and its variation are used in many sports classes. All variations support the venous blood stream and relieve the legs. Make sure that you put a bolster in the right position under your shoulders, and save your neck from a harsh bend.

Notes of Caution and Contraindications

Shoulder stands are not recommended for people who suffer from pain in the cervical vertebrae, high blood pressure, or eye or ear conditions.

Alignments

Place the bolster on top of the mat and under the shoulder. The edge of the bolster is parallel to the edge of the shoulders. The spinal column is stretched out as in the upright stance. The pelvis is in an upright position with muscles tightened.

What to Do

- Place your mat at a right angle to a wall. Put a folded blanket on your mat. Lie down on your back with your shoulders at the edge of the folded blanket and your knees bent. Place both your feet hip width apart on the ground. Stretch out your arms at the side of your body. Both palms are facing downward.
- Exhaling, bring your knees to your chest and stretch your legs.
- Inhaling, roll your spine upward and lift your hips and torso. To support the lifting, place your hands at the top of your hips. You can either do the complete stretch during one inhalation, or raise legs and torso in a couple of moves, resting during exhalations.

- To stabilize and simplify the posture, place your feet against a wall. Your lower legs are parallel to the floor.

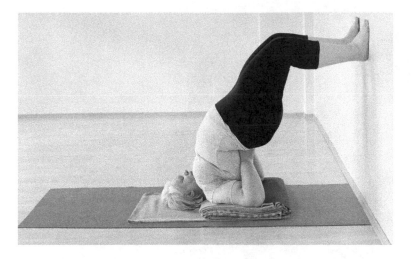

- Keep the position for six complete inhalations and exhalations.
- To get out of the posture, move your feet downward at the wall while exhaling.
- Lower your spine vertebra by vertebra. Place your feet on the ground, and put your hands and arms alongside your body.
- Feel the effects of the inversion. You may close your eyes if you like to do so.

Variation as a Free-Standing Shoulder Stand

- Come into the shoulder stand using a wall as a prop.
- Inhaling, stretch your right leg.

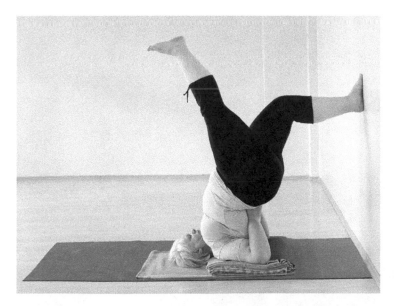

- Exhaling, pause and make sure you are maintaining your stability.
- Inhaling, stretch your left leg and come into the full posture.

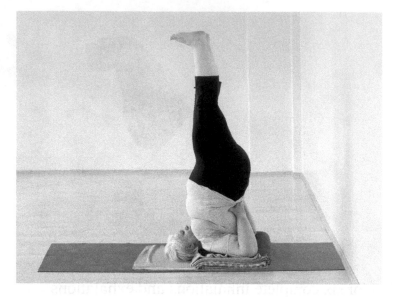

- Keep the position for six complete inhalations and exhalations.
- To get out of the posture: Exhaling, place your feet—one at a time—back on the wall. Pause on an inhalation.
- Exhaling, move your feet downward on the wall.
- Lower your spine vertebra by vertebra. Place your feet on the ground, and put your hands and arms alongside your body.
- Feel the effects of the inversion. You may close your eyes if it feels comfortable.

LEGS UP THE WALL

Purposes

Legs up the wall is recommended if you want to relieve pain in your legs and feet. In this posture, you benefit from an inversion even if you suffer from pain in your cervical vertebrae.

Notes of Caution and Contraindications

Put a cushion under your head if you suffer from high blood pressure or eye or ear conditions.

Alignments

Do not hyperextend your knees. Use blankets to bolster your back, and place your head on a cushion if it feels more comfortable and helps you to relax.

What to Do

- Place your mat at a right angle to a wall. Put a folded blanket on your mat. Sit upright with bent knees and your right shoulder alongside a wall.
- With an inhalation, slowly rotate, bending your torso backward and your legs upward against the wall.

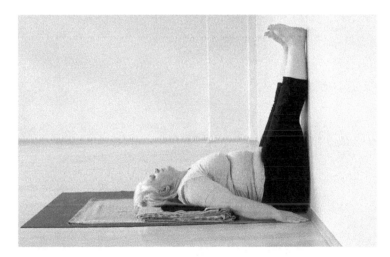

- Stretch your spine, and place your arms alongside your body.
- Place your heels against the wall.
- Keep the posture for at least six complete inhalations and exhalations.
- Exhaling, bend your knees and roll to the side.
- Inhaling, slowly roll your torso upward.
- Rest with your back against the wall, and feel the effects of the exercise.
- Close your eyes if it feels comfortable.

Eye Exercises

Eye exercises are very beneficial, increasing blood circulation, relaxing eyes and body, and enhancing the ability to concentrate. They also help maintain good eyesight and can compensate for age-related vision loss. Exercising the eyes for just a few minutes every day improves the ability of the ocular muscles to adapt to the loss of flexibility that happens as we age. Eye exercises also relieve itchy, burning eyes by helping the eyes to remain moist.

I recommend including the following three exercises in a daily yoga routine (see also Part IV).

FOCUS NEAR AND FAR

Purposes

Focus near and far is a workout for the eye muscles. Eye muscles need to be exercised in order to stay flexible and strong like all other muscles. By focusing on objects at the same distance every day, for example, while working at the computer, reading, or watching TV, we weaken our eye muscles over time in the same way that we weaken our back and leg muscles by sitting for extended periods of time.

Notes of Caution and Contraindications

There are no contraindications for this exercise. If you have serious eye problems such as glaucoma or macular degeneration, talk to your doctor about the following exercises.

Alignments

If you normally wear glasses, take them off while you are exercising. Actively alternate your focus on close and distant objects.

What to Do

- Sit upright on a chair. If you do the eye exercises sitting on a mat, come into the free seat with knees bent. To be able to exercise for a couple of minutes, make sure that you are in a comfortable posture.
- Extend one arm to eye level and make a fist with your thumb up.
- Look at the tip of your nose and breathe in and out.
- Look at your thumbnail and breathe in and out.

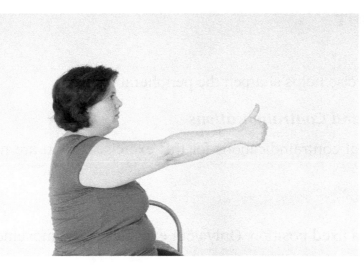

- Look at an object close by and breathe in and out.
- Look at an object in the distance and breathe in and out.
- Next, during a complete inhalation and exhalation, no longer lock your eyes at an object, and just look into the sky or ahead of you.
- Repeat each step in reverse order until you are looking at your nose again.
- Restart the cycle. Do the complete exercise six times.
- Keep to a steady breathing rhythm that matches the pace of your movements.

THE LYING EIGHT

Purposes

The lying eight exercise helps sharpen the peripheral vision.

Notes of Caution and Contraindications

There are no general contraindications for this exercise. If you are not sure, talk to your doctor.

Alignments

Keep your head in a fixed position. Only your eyes follow the movements of your thumb.

What to Do

- Sit upright on a chair. If you are exercising on a mat, come into the free seat with knees bent. To be able to exercise for a couple of minutes, make sure that you are in a comfortable posture.
- Extend your right arm to eye level, make a fist, and keep your thumb up. Focus on your thumbnail with both eyes. Hold your head in a fixed position and do not move it. Only the eyes move during this exercise as they focus on and follow the movements of your thumb.

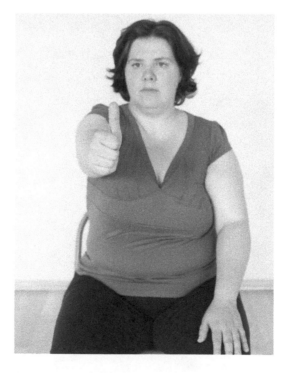

- Slowly raise your stretched out arm directing it upward.
- Move your arm along the upper right half of your peripheral view.

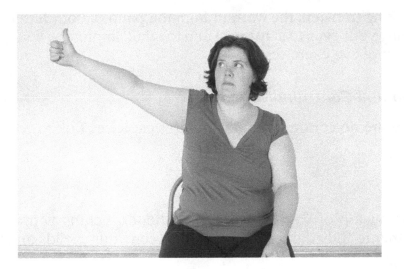

- Continue moving it completely to the right to the point where your thumbnail is still visible.
- Slowly continue the move of your stretched arm downward along the lower right half of your peripheral view.

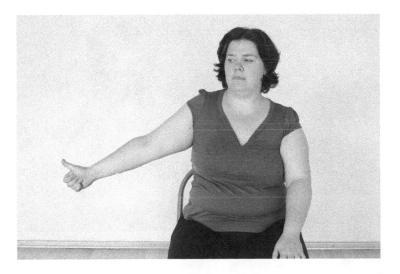

- Proceed until moving back to the starting position.
- Lower your right arm, bring your left arm up, and do the same exercise to the left side.
- Repeat the exercise three times to each side.
- Keep a steady breathing rhythm that matches the pace of your movements.

CUPPING AND BLINKING

Purposes

Cupping and blinking transfers the warmth from the palm of your hands to your eyes and eye sockets, helping your eyes to stay moist and to relax, improving your vision. It is a good way to close the set of eye exercises.

Notes of Caution and Contraindications

Once again: There are no contraindications for this exercise. Talk to your doctor if you are not sure.

Alignments

Place your palms on top of your closed eyes without touching your eyelids. Bring your hands close together to fully darken the space between your eyelids and your palms.

What to Do

- Sit upright on a chair or on a mat.
- Rub your hands forcefully together until you sense the warmth.

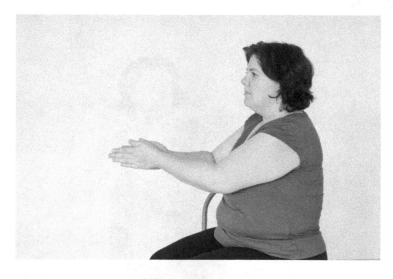

■ Completely cover your closed eyes with your palms—the fingers are upright against the front of your face. Without any contact between your palms and your eyelids, feel the warmth being transferred, and completely relax your eyes.

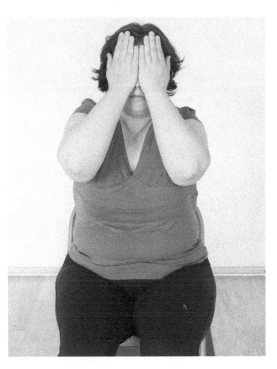

■ After a while, remove your palms from your eyes, relax your arms, and keep your eyes closed.
■ Start blinking with your eyelids, changing from quick blinks to slower blinks.
■ Open your eyes, relax your whole body, and feel the effects.

Pranayama

Calm, rhythmic breathing techniques, called pranayama, are an essential element of yoga. They enhance the oxygen level in the blood, increasing muscle power and mental power. Pranayama also helps to relieve emotional tension and stress. Nostril breathing is generally performed while you do yoga and is the basis for all pranayama. It is vital that you do not underestimate its effect.

ALTERNATE NOSTRIL BREATHING

Purposes

This alternate nostril breathing exercise immediately widens the bronchial tubes, promotes even breathing, relaxes the body, calms the mind, and increases awareness. You will slowly develop a steady breathing rhythm composed of regular, complete inhalations and exhalations. When alternate nostril breathing is practiced regularly, you will notice if there are differences between your inhalations and exhalations. For some, it is easy to inhale fully but difficult to exhale completely, while for others it is the other way around. People with asthma will benefit greatly from this technique. Another great plus: It can be done almost anywhere.

Notes of Caution and Contraindications

There are no general contraindications for this exercise. Practice with care and consciousness to feel its full benefit. Stop the exercise if you feel dizzy.

Alignments

Sit upright and relax. Use a bolster or table to support your working hand and arm if you like.

What to Do

- Sit on a chair or get into a comfortable position on your mat.
- Bend the index finger, middle finger, and ring finger of your right hand, and stretch out your thumb and little finger.
- Place your right thumb next to your right nostril and your right little finger next to the left nostril. Either place your bent arm on a table, or hold it comfortably in front of your body so that it is not pushing on your thorax and is not blocking your breathing.
- To begin, first breathe out deeply through both nostrils.

■ Close your right nostril with your thumb, and slowly breathe in through your left nostril.

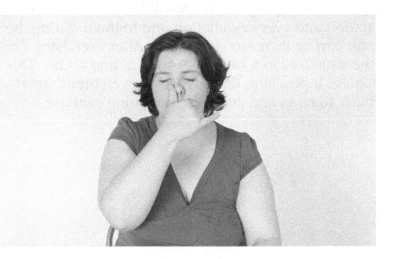

■ Close the left nostril with your little finger and slowly breathe out completely through the right nostril.

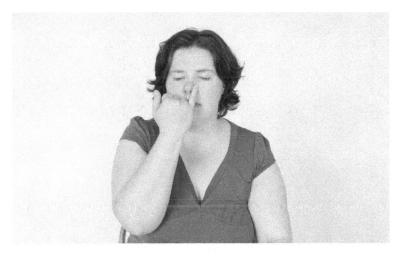

■ Slowly breathe in again through the right nostril. Close your right nostril with your thumb, and slowly breathe out again through the left nostril.

■ Repeat the alternate nostril breathing for at least six complete breath cycles.

■ Finally, lower your hand, and breathe in and out through both your nostrils. Feel the calming effects. Keep your eyes closed if it feels comfortable.

Variation with Different Breathing Rhythms

To achieve as even a breathing rhythm as possible, you can count to six in your mind between every inhalation and every exhalation and to three during the breaks in between. Your volume of breath can be increased with time. After exercising like this for some time, you can carry out the exercises in a ratio of 8:4, 10:5, and so on. This depends, however, on your ability to achieve a pleasant, thorough, and even breathing rhythm. Stop counting if it reduces your ability to relax and enjoy the breathing exercise.

TIGER BREATHING

Purposes

Tiger breathing enhances awareness of your spine and widens the space between your vertebrae. In addition, it synchronizes breathing and movement. If you can bend and stretch your spine consciously, you can check and correct your posture throughout the day.

Notes of Caution and Contraindications

There are no contraindications. Use a bolster under your knees and ankles (if necessary) to feel comfortable during the whole exercise.

Alignments

Place your wrists under your shoulders and your knees under your hip joints. Make sure that you do not block your elbows.

What to Do

- Come into the kneeling posture.
- With an inhalation, bend forward until your hands touch the floor (on all fours).
- Make sure that your wrists are under your shoulders and that your knees are under your hip joints. These alignments help you to exercise without hurting your joints.

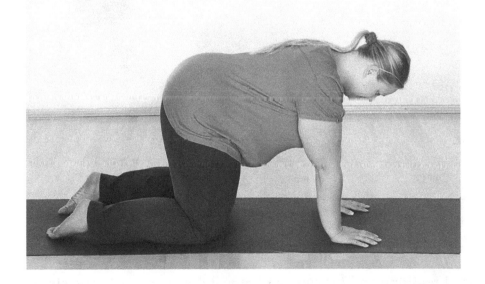

■ On the exhalation, bend your spine, vertebra by vertebra, starting at your tailbone and moving all the way up through the lumbar, thoracic, and cervical spine. Bow your head last.

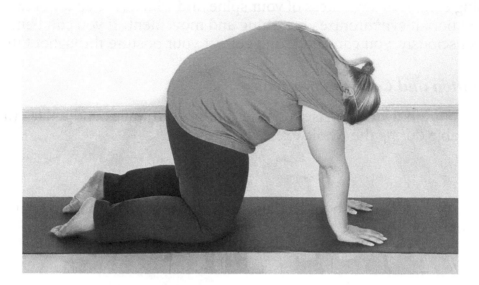

■ On the inhalation, stretch your spine, vertebra by vertebra, starting at your tailbone and moving all the way up through the lumbar, thoracic, and cervical spine. Lift your head last.

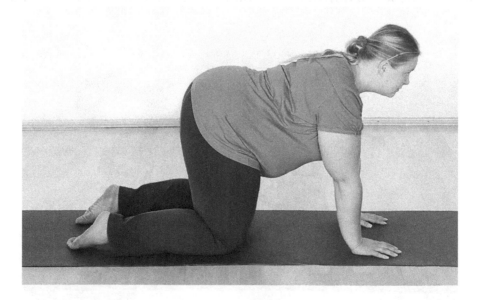

■ Synchronize breathing and moving, and repeat the exercise during six complete inhalations and exhalations.
■ Inhaling, get back into the kneeling posture again. Place your fingers on top of your thighs and relax. Feel the effects with your eyes closed if it feels comfortable.

CAMEL POSTURE

Purposes

The camel posture widens the chest and expands breathing capacity. It also deepens breathing by lowering the diaphragm. It strengthens shoulder and arm muscles as well as thigh and belly muscles, and it flexes the back.

Notes of Caution and Contraindications

The vigorous breathing combined with a lift of the torso can influence blood circulation. If you feel dizzy, get back into the starting position, or lie down on your back with knees bent or legs up against the wall.

Alignments

Keep your thighs in an upright position while you are bending backward.

■ Come into the kneeling posture. Let your arms hang at the side of your body.

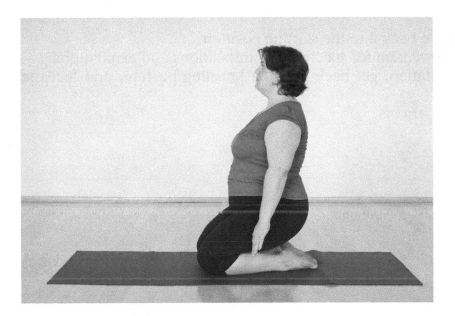

■ Inhaling, rise on your knees and open your arms to the side. Make sure that your thighs are in an upright position and your pubic bone is pushing forward.

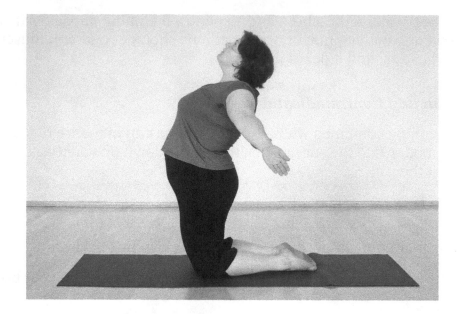

■ Exhaling, move back into the starting position.
■ Repeat the movement for six complete inhalations and exhalations.
■ With an exhalation, get back into the kneeling posture, and feel the effects of the exercise.

GREAT GESTURE

Purposes

Great gesture is performed in a kneeling position, but it is also possible to do it in an upright standing position. This exercise flexes neck and shoulder muscles and enlarges the breathing space.

Notes of Caution and Contraindications

This vigorous movement of the needs some practice. Great gesture is not recommended for people with high blood pressure or eye or ear conditions. Stop the exercise if you feel dizzy.

Alignments

Be gentle with your shoulder joints, and start with small movements. Use a bolster if it feels more comfortable.

What to Do

- Come into the kneeling posture.

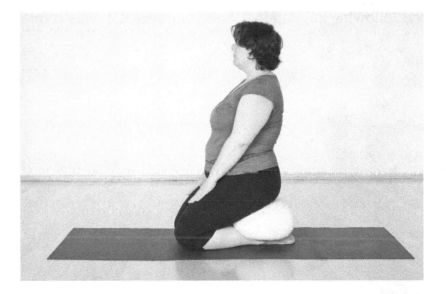

- Stretch out your arms and move them backward. Bring your hands together behind your back and cross your fingers—your palms should be facing your back.
- Inhale through your nose in this position.

■ Exhaling through your nose, bend forward and simultaneously lift your arms three times. (Make sure that you do not inhale in-between movements and that you use the movement of your arms to exhale entirely.)

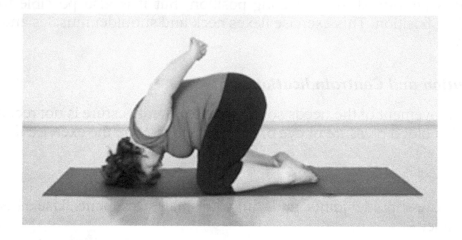

■ Inhaling, gently stretch out your neck, and lift your stretched-out torso into the starting position.
■ Repeat the movements during six complete inhalations and exhalations.
■ Finally, keep the kneeling posture, and feel the effects of the stretch and the strong exhalation and following inhalation. Close your eyes if it feels comfortable.

15

Relaxing Postures

The following two yoga postures will help you become aware of the effects your yoga practice has had on your body, breathing, thoughts, and feelings.

KAYA KRIYA

Purposes

Kaya kriya is an exercise that develops your awareness through conscious breathing and moving. It focuses your attention, relaxes body and mind, and provides a gentle mobilization of joints.

Notes of Caution and Contraindications

There are no contraindications for kaya kriya. If it feels more comfortable or if you want to practice with your head above heart level, use a bolster.

Alignments

Remember to stretch your neck, and do not bow your head while turning it. Lift your head a little to prevent bowing.

What to Do

- Lie on your back. Stretch your entire spine. Your neck is stretched, and your chin is lowered toward your sternum. Your eyes can be closed, and your face and mouth muscles are relaxed. Your shoulders are relaxed and lie flat on the mat. Your arms lie by the sides of your body. Place your legs a few inches apart. Your big toes should touch if you rotate your feet.

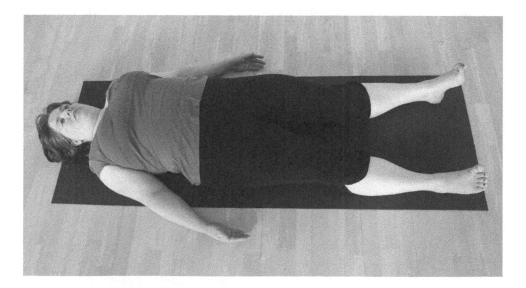

■ Inhaling, rotate your feet inward until your big toes touch, rotate your arms outward away from your sides, and turn your head to the right. Make sure that you do not bow your head at the same time.

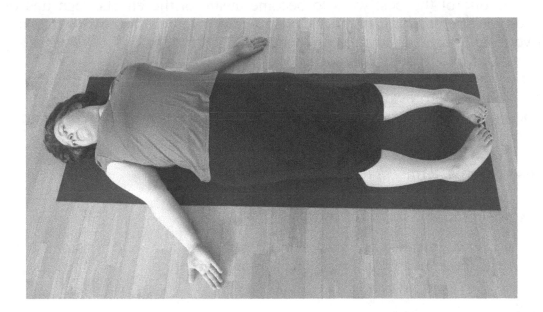

■ Exhaling, rotate your feet outward, rotate your arms toward your sides, and turn your head to the left.

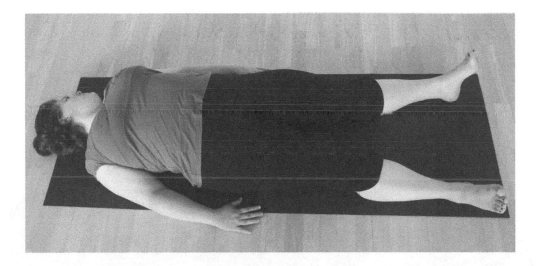

■ Repeat the movements for six complete inhalations and exhalations.
■ Return to the starting position. Your arms lie by the sides of your body with the palms of the hands facing the ceiling. Your feet are rotated outward. Feel the effects of kaya kriya.

YOGA NIDRA

Purposes

Yoga nidra is one of the best ways to become aware of the effects yoga has on different parts of your body. You can either develop your own way of moving your awareness through your body or be guided by a teacher (either in a class or at home using a CD). There are advantages to both methods.

Practicing on your own can be helpful if you have trouble falling asleep. Yoga nidra can be practiced in bed to provide a good sleep. However, it requires regular practice and the development of a rhythm as you move your attention from body part to body part. Bringing the awareness toward a certain part of the body while listening to a voice is very relaxing. Doing yoga nidra this way can give you the feeling of being directly connected to your body without using words, terms, or images.

Notes of Caution and Contraindications

There are no contraindications for yoga nidra. Place your head on a bolster if you want to keep your head above heart level, or if it feels more comfortable.

Alignments

There is no right way of doing yoga nidra; just find a way that works best for you.

What to Do

- Stretch out lying on your back (see shanti asana, Chapter 3).

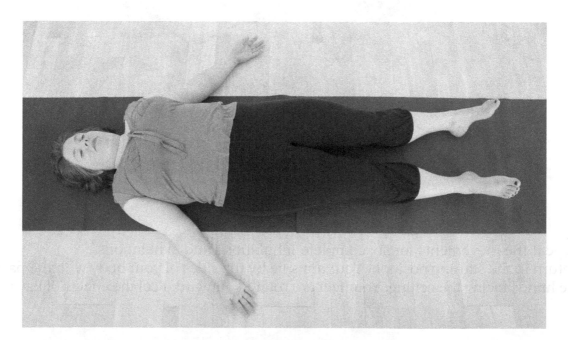

- Bring your attention to your left feet, your left sole, your left ankle, your left lower leg, your left knee, your left thigh, your left hip joint.
- Bring your attention to your right foot, your right sole, your right ankle, your right lower leg, your right knee, your right thigh, your right hip joint.
- Bring your attention to your left hand, your left palm, your left wrist, your left forearm, your left ellbow, your left upper arm, your left shoulder joint.
- Bring your attention to your right hand, your right palm, your right wrist, your right forearm, your right ellbow, your right upper arm, your right shoulder joint.
- Bring your attention to the back of your head where it lies on the mat, to your forehead, to the front of your body, your left brow, your right brow, your left eye, your right eye, the tip of your nose, your upper lip, your lower lip, the tip of your chin.
- Bring your attention to your belly, observing how it moves up and down. Keep your attention on your belly for a couple of inhalations and exhalations.
- If you have practiced yoga nidra in bed, you may feel relaxed and ready to sleep.
- If you want to get out of the posture, completely inhale and exhale through your nose a couple of times.
- Make small movements with your toes and fingers, with your feet and hands, with your legs and arms. Stretch your body if it feels good.
- Get up into a seated posture, and feel the effects of yoga nidra with your eyes closed.

16

Awareness and Meditation

If you have experienced calm and relaxing moments during your yoga practice and want to extend them, it is vital to develop a steady practice of meditation.

While practicing yoga postures, you are focused on your alignment and breath, which helps you relax by shifting the focus of your thinking. At the end of a session, your mind is calm. Meditative exercises work similarly to get you into a quiet, relaxed mood.

Meditation requires practice before you can benefit fully from its positive effects on body and mind. There is no right way to move from working on your body to working on your meditative practice, but I encourage you to incorporate meditation into your daily practice. To develop your abilities to meditate, it is helpful to concentrate on your progress and honor the relaxing affects and the moments that provide a positive feeling. People suffering from delusions should not meditate. Check with your doctor, if you are not sure.

Meditating involves being open-minded, conscious, and relaxed. If you've never meditated before, it may be helpful to compare it to the experiences of being awake and being asleep as in the below chart:

Qualities → State of awareness ↓	Being open-minded	Being conscious	Being relaxed
Sleeping	Yes Anything might happen in our dreams.	No Sleeping is the opposite of being conscious.	Yes and No A good sleep is relaxing, but sleep can also be stressful and intimidating: People chew on their teeth while sleeping or suddenly wake up from fearful dreams.
Being awake	Yes and No Being open-minded depends on the issue, the way we are approached, and our individual resources such as strength and the ability to relax.	Yes We ignore the moments of absentmindedness and think of them as exceptions.	Yes and No This book is meant to help you be relaxed in stressful situations. Unfortunately, as long as we live, we always experience situations and moments that are stressful and that we can hardly cope with.
Meditating	Yes Being able to meditate enables us to open up to thoughts and feelings.	Yes Most obviously, we are conscious in active forms of meditation: asana, pranayama, reciting or singing mantras, but also while meditating and listening to sounds, focusing on objects, inner pictures, or our own breathing.	Yes Meditation leads to a profound state of tranquility and relaxation.

WALKING MEDITATION

Walking meditation is a good way to withdraw your attention from outside stimuli. As you walk, concentrate on the various sensations you feel—from the pressure on the soles of your feet, the movement of your knees, hips, and spine to the warmth of your hands. For best results, practice in a quiet space, such as a park, even a large room.

The easiest way to find out if walking is an effective form of mediation for you is to practice and experience it. If you already know you enjoy walking, find a private place, like a short path around your yard. Start with five minutes, and slowly extend the time with each practice. As you walk, focus on every aspect of the activity, including how your joints feel, which parts of your body are relaxed, and which are active. Notice how long you can keep your attention focused, and celebrate your new ability.

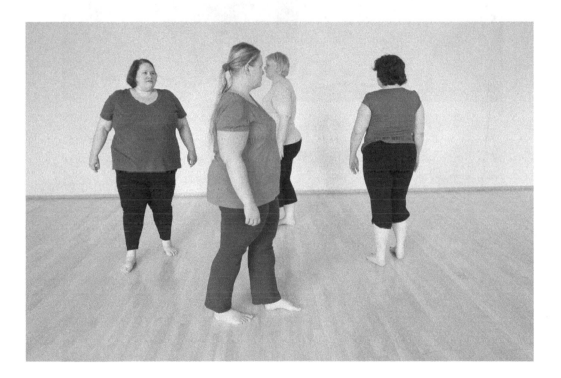

MEDITATION ON YOUR BODY

Focusing your attention on your body and praising it for the work it does to sustain you ever day is another simple yet powerful way to meditate. Begin either with your feet or head, and work your way up or down your body. For example, you may wish to start with the ears that help you listen and connect with others or your feet that support you every day. You can also concentrate on and honor one organ or one part of your body.

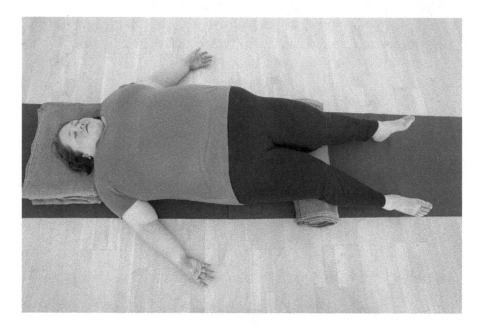

MANTRA MEDITATION

A mantra can be a syllable, a word, a line, a poem, or a song. You can choose a single word in English that means something important to you, such as stamina, love, or confidence or a word in Sanskrit, such as ananda (bliss), jaya (victory), or shanty (peace). You can also choose a statement like *give it a try* or *action brings success*. Whatever you choose, recite it over and over, aloud or in your mind, with patience and resolution.

You may be familiar with the most famous yoga mantra, "OM." OM has many interpretations, and, if you choose to use it, you may choose one that suits your needs and beliefs. Part of the appeal of OM is, undoubtedly, that it sounds good and can be recited or sung alone (either in your mind or aloud) and in groups.

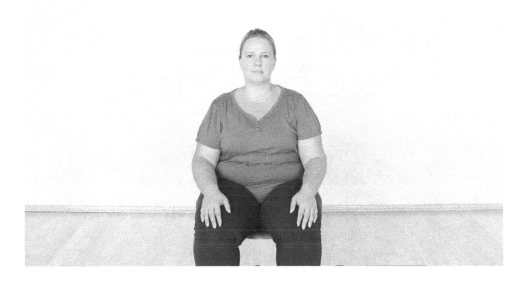

SOUND MEDITATION

Singing bowls, bells, and cymbals have been used in yoga meditation for centuries. Made of metal or glass, they produce various tones—high, low, short, and long—when hitting the bowl with a mallet or circling the mallet around the rim of a bowl. Sound meditation comes by concentrating for as long as possible on the sound produced. You do not need to buy any specialized instruments to practice sound meditation. Use a glass bowl or glass from your cupboard. Or, hum or sing a favorite tune and concentrate on the sound. Become aware of how long you can focus your mind on the sound, then refocus as the sound fades.

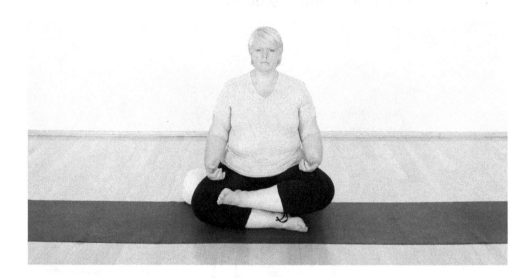

VISUAL MEDITATION

As the name suggests, visual meditation requires focusing attention on a single object. In many representations of yoga, a candle is used, but any photo, painting, written word, or object will do, real or imagined. Concentrate on the object for as long as possible. Become aware of how long you are able to maintain this attention.

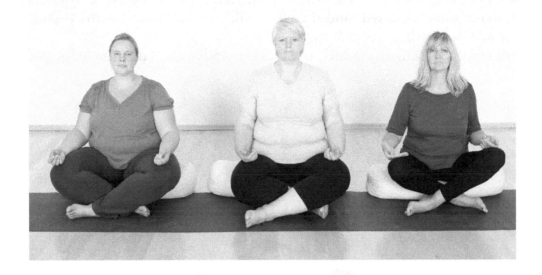

SILENCE IN THE STREAM OF YOUR THOUGHTS

Silence in the stream of your thoughts is intended to give your thoughts a break. We are usually bombarded by an overwhelming amount of information—data, appointments, contacts, and conversations. It can be difficult to discriminate between what is important and what is not. Through the practice of meditation, you can learn to concentrate on a feeling, sound, or photo and experience a profound pause in the stream of your thoughts. Experiment with the methods I have described to determine which one works best for you. As you gain experience, you will find it easy to slide into a state in which you are able to extend the space in between your thoughts.

Be patient with yourself, enjoy each meditation, and always acknowledge your progress.

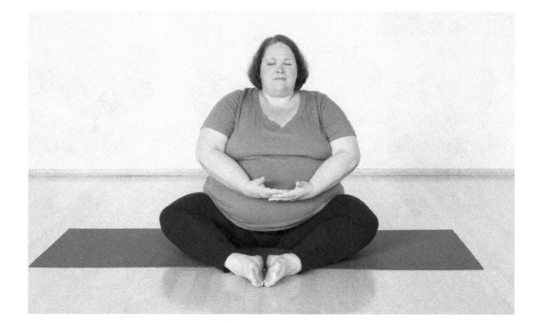

PART III

POSTURES IN FLOWING

MOTION

Practicing yoga in flowing motion—moving into and out of a posture—enhances your mobility. Before you try to do the following combinations of postures, you should have practiced each posture for some time.

Yoga done in flowing motion is very popular in yoga classes. If you decide to attend a class, it is important to find a teacher who understands your individual needs. For some people, it is difficult to flow from one posture into the other, whereas for others, it is difficult to stay in a posture for a long time. Find the teacher and class that support your personal well-being.

Swinging Arms

The following combination of yoga postures in motion is a workout for your arms that will also challenge your sense of balance as you move from one posture into the other.

There are no general contraindications for this set of postures.

POSTURE 1: TRIANGLE IN MOTION

Purposes

The triangle in motion stretches your flank muscles, arms, and hands.

Notes of Caution and Contraindications

This modified version of the triangle posture gives you a gentle stretch and has no general contraindications.

Alignments

It is vital to exercise to the side and stretch the flanks.

What to Do

- Come into the upright standing posture.
- Shift your weight to your left foot.
- Inhaling, move your right foot in front of your left foot, move your right arm in front of your belly (bend your right hand), lift your left arm (bend your left hand), and turn your head to the right.

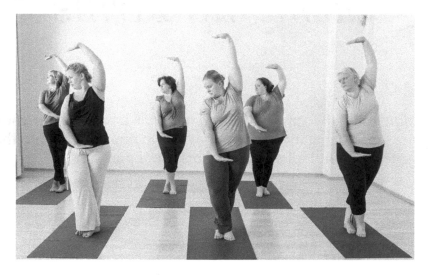

- Pause with an exhalation.
- Inhaling, move your left foot in front of your right foot, move your left arm in front of your belly (bend your left hand), lift your right arm (bend your right hand), and turn your head to the left.
- Pause with an exhalation.
- Repeat the movements during six complete inhalations and exhalations.
- Continue with posture 2.

POSTURE 2: ARM LIFT

Purposes

The arm lift mobilizes the shoulder joints, strengthens arm and shoulder muscles, and improves arm coordination.

Notes of Caution and Contraindications

These movements have no general contraindications.

Alignments

Evenly distribute your weight on your soles. Stretch your arms, and make sure your palms face each other.

What to Do

- Continue from triangle in motion.
- Inhaling, stretch both arms over your head (palms facing each other).

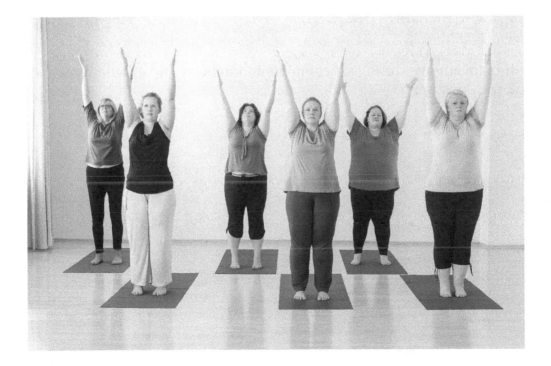

- Exhaling, lower your arms, and place your hands on your belly (fold one arm over the other).

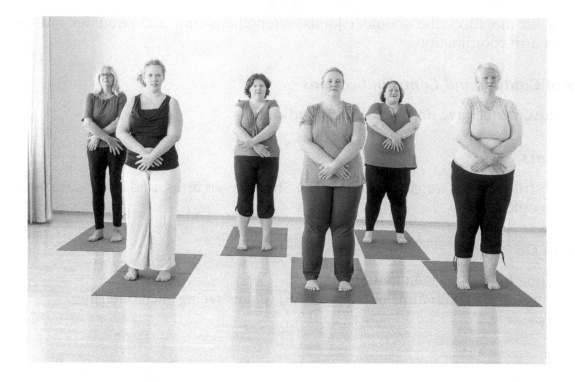

- Repeat the movements during six complete inhalations and exhalations.
- Continue with posture 3.

POSTURE 3: ARM ROTATION

Purposes

Arm rotations counter poor posture, mobilize shoulder joints, and strengthen arm muscles.

Notes of Caution and Contraindications

These rotations have no general contraindications.

Alignments

Keep your arms at shoulder height. Make sure that you are raising just your arms, not your shoulders.

What to Do

- Continue from arm lift (posture 2).
- Inhaling, lift both arms sideways to shoulder height.
- Exhaling, rotate your stretched arms backward until your palms are facing downward.

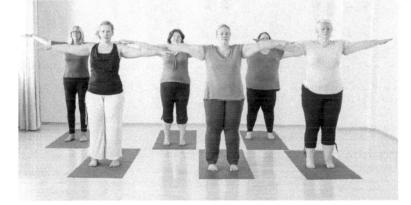

- Inhaling, rotate your stretched arms forward until your palms are facing upward.

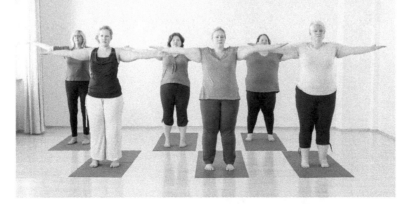

- Repeat the rotations during six complete inhalations and exhalations.
- Continue with the next posture, repeating the arm lift (posture 2).

185

POSTURE 4: REPEAT POSTURE 2, ARM LIFT

For notes of caution and alignments, see posture 2.

What to Do

- Continue from arm rotation (posture 3).
- With an inhalation, stretch both arms over your head (palms facing each other).

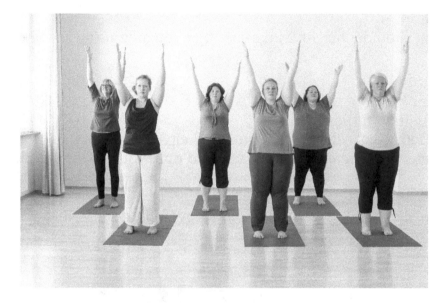

- Continue with posture 5.

POSTURE 5: FOLDED HANDS

Purposes

This is a very effective exercise for expanding the chest, strengthening the shoulder and arm muscles, and stretching the complete upper torso from the waist to the neck.

Notes of Caution and Contraindications

There are no general contraindications for this posture.

Alignments

Push your palms together. Stretch your neck with your chin parallel to the floor. Relax your shoulders.

What to Do

- Continue from arm lift (posture 4).
- Exhaling, lower your arms.
- Inhaling, bring your palms together at the height of your chest.
- Exhaling, push your hands together and relax your shoulders.
- Keep the posture for six complete inhalations and exhalations.

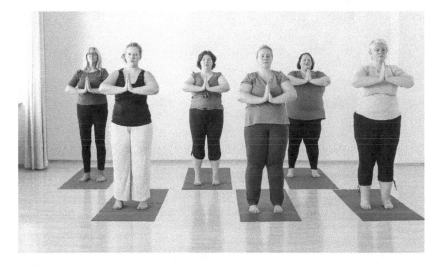

- Finally, lower your arms on an exhale. Feel the effects of the whole set of postures in motion with your eyes closed if it feels comfortable.

18

Fancy Leg and Footwork

This series of postures provides an energetic workout for your legs and feet. It is easier to enjoy the exercise if you have strengthened your leg and foot muscles by regularly practicing the standing postures such as the hero.

There are no general contraindications for this set of postures.

POSTURE 1: CHAIR POSTURE WITH FOLDED HANDS

Purposes

This posture expands your chest muscles, strengthens the thigh, arm, and leg muscles, and mobilizes your shoulder, hip, and knee joints.

Notes of Caution and Contraindications

There are no general contraindications for this posture.

Alignments

To support your knee joints, exercise with knees and ankles in line (knees exactly over ankles).

What to Do

- You can either continue from folded arms (chapter 17, posture 5) or start in an upright standing posture.
- Exhaling, push your palms together at the height of your chest. Make sure your shoulders are relaxed.
- Inhaling, concentrate on your legs and feet.
- Exhaling, release your hips back as though you are going to sit.
- Inhaling, stretch your legs until you are standing in an upright position.
- Repeat the bending and stretching of your knees during six complete inhalations and exhalations.

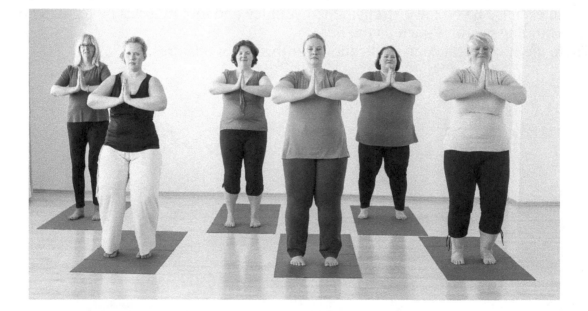

POSTURE 2: CHAIR POSTURE WITH SPLAYED FINGERS

Purposes

This posture is a balancing asana that also strengthens your leg and foot muscles.

Notes of Caution and Contraindications

There are no general contraindications for this posture.

Alignments

To support your knee joints, exercise with knees and ankles in line (knees exactly over ankles).

What to Do

- Continue from chair posture with folded hands. Exhaling, bend your knees.
- Inhaling, stretch your arms, bend your wrists, and splay your fingers.
- Keep the posture for six complete inhalations and exhalations.
- Continue with posture 3.

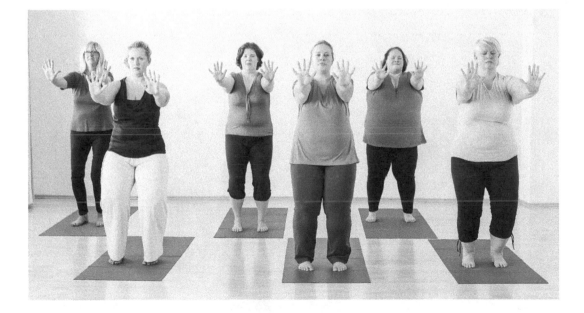

POSTURE 3: CHAIR POSTURE WITH OUTSTRETCHED ARMS

Purposes

This posture is meant to train your thigh and arm muscles.

Notes of Caution and Contraindications

There are no general contraindications for this posture.

Alignments

Exercising in the chair posture is very demanding. Check the alignment of your knees and ankles. Always support your knee joints by exercising with knees and ankles in line (knees exactly over ankles). Make sure that you stay concentrated, and do not harm your knee joints.

What to Do

- Continue from chair posture with splayed fingers (posture 2).
- Inhaling, lower your hands and stretch your wrist. Rotate your outstretched arms until your palms are facing each other.
- Keep the posture for six complete inhalations and exhalations.
- Continue with posture 4.

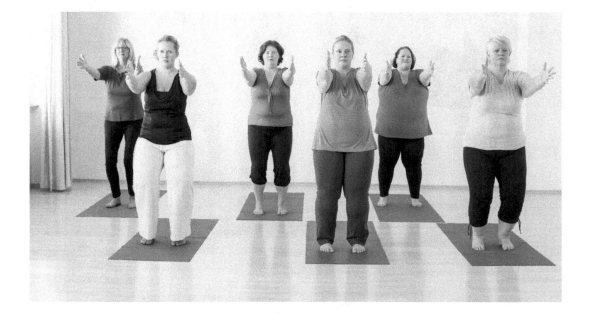

POSTURE 4: FORWARD BOW WITH STRETCHED KNEES

Purposes

The forward bow is a relaxing counterpose. After exercising with bent knees and an upright torso, you will now bow your torso and stretch your knees.

Notes of Caution and Contraindications

If you suffer from high blood pressure or eye and ear conditions, do not lower your head below heart level.

Alignments

Fully relax your torso. Use a block if you cannot relax in a forward bend. Do not lock your knee joints; stretch your knees without overdoing it. Do not forcefully bring your hands to the mat. Use a prop if necessary.

What to Do

- Continue from chair posture with stretched out arms.
- Exhaling, lower your outstretched arms and your torso until your hands meet with the mat or blocks. Inhaling, moderately stretch your legs. Make sure that this posture feels comfortable and relaxing.
- Keep the posture for six complete inhalations and exhalations.
- Inhaling, slowly roll up your torso vertebra by vertebra until you are standing in an upright posture.
- Feel the effects of the set of postures in motion with your eyes closed if it feels comfortable to you.

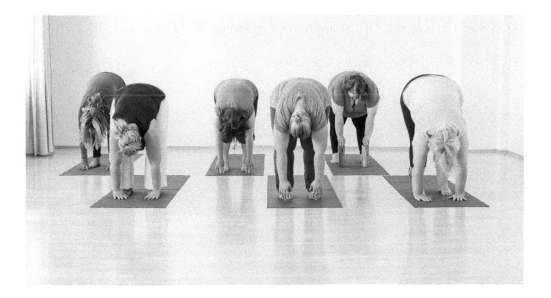

19

Arm and Leg Coordination

The following combination is playful and demanding, requiring a strong sense of balance and coordination.

"What I like best about our group? There is a certain humor in handling problems and respect for one another. Nobody is annoyed, if one of us has problems with a posture."

—Anika

POSTURE 1: HERO 2

Purposes

The hero 2 posture is a very energetic posture that will boost your mood. It strengthens the foot, leg, and spine muscles and will challenge your sense of balance.

Notes of Caution and Contraindications

There are no general contraindications. Be gentle with your knees and keep knees and ankles in line.

Alignments

Stretch your spine and keep your torso centered. Your pelvis and your forward-pointing foot are in line. Keep your arms stretched and at shoulder height. This posture is perfect and most beneficial for your knees if your ankles are under your knees.

What to Do

- Start in an upright standing posture with your left foot pointing forward and your right foot pointing inward. Your hands rest on your pelvis.
- Exhaling, lower your torso until your left leg is bent with your left knee over the ankle of your left foot.

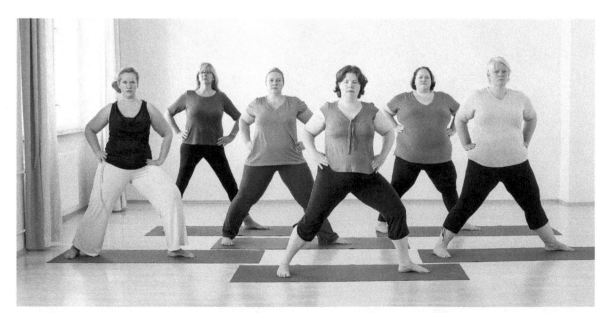

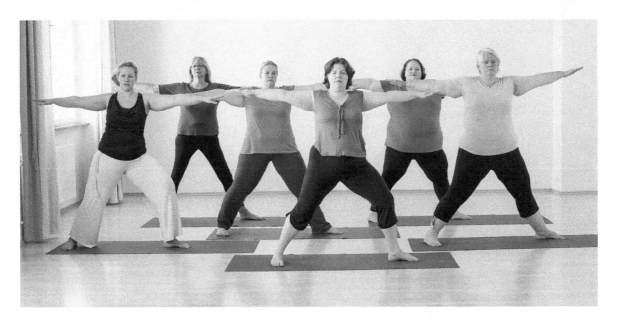

- Inhaling, lift your arms to shoulder level. Make sure that your body is centered.
- Exhaling, lower your right arm and lift your left arm.

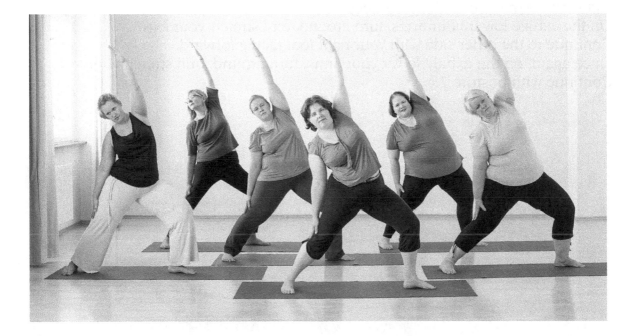

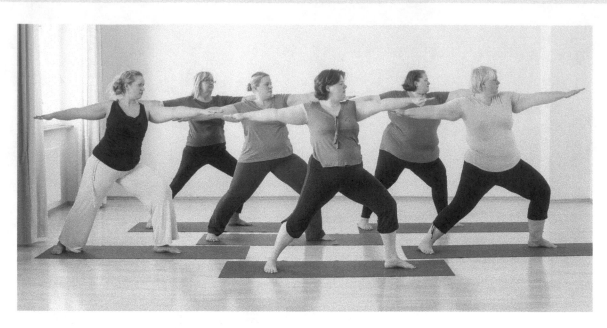

- ■ Keep the posture during six complete inhalations and exhalations.
- ■ Inhaling, stretch your arms at shoulder height.
- ■ Exhaling, turn your head to the left.
- ■ Keep the posture during six complete inhalations and exhalations. The posture is perfect if both arms are at shoulder height.
- ■ On the exhale lower your arms, turn around, and stretch your legs.
- ■ Continue to the other side with your right foot facing forward.
- ■ Once again, on the exhale lower your arms, turn around, and stretch your legs.
- ■ Continue with posture 2.

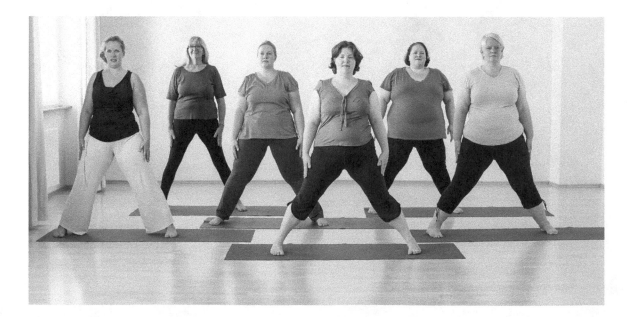

POSTURE 2: FOLDED ARMS IN STANDING POSITION

Purposes

This posture is more relaxing than hero 2 and improves your arm coordination while strengthening your arm and shoulder muscles.

Notes of Caution and Contraindications

There are no general contraindications.

Alignments

Keep your arms stretched out and relax your shoulders.

What to Do

- Continue from the hero 2 posture.
- Inhaling, lift your arms over the side to shoulder height.

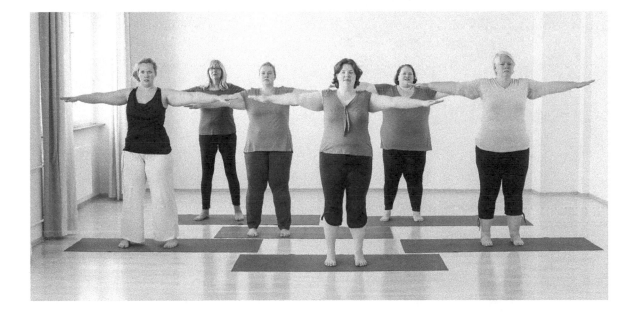

- Exhaling, fold your left arm over your right arm.
- Inhaling, open your arms at shoulder height.
- Exhaling, fold your right arm over your left arm.
- Continue with posture 3.

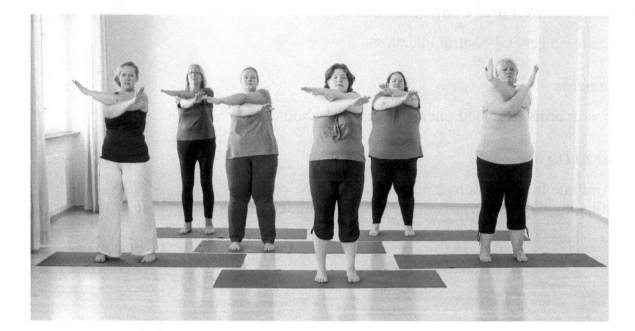

POSTURE 3: CROSSED LEGS AND FOLDED HANDS

Purposes

This exercise concludes this combination of yoga postures in motion. Once again, you will challenge your coordination, enhance your stability, and strengthen your chest, flank, and thigh muscles.

Notes of Caution and Contraindications

There are no general contraindications.

Alignments

Relax your shoulders. If you have a good sense of balance, close your eyes.

What to Do

- Continue from the folded arms in standing position.
- Exhaling, lower your arms.
- Inhaling, lift your left foot, cross it over your right foot, and place your left foot on the mat. At the same time bend your arms and push your palms together at chest height.
- Keep the posture for six complete inhalations and exhalations.
- Continue to the other side.
- Finally, exhaling, lower your arms and come into the upright standing position. Feel the effects of the whole set of postures in motion. Close your eyes if you like.

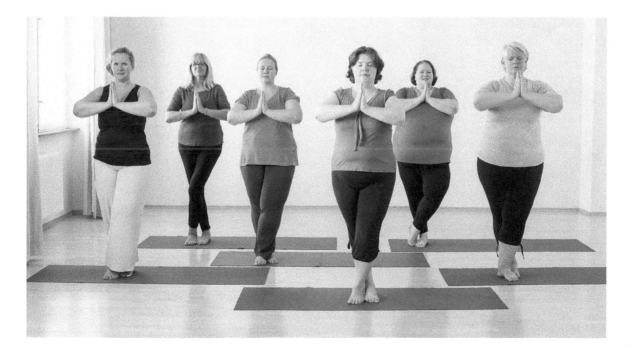

PART
IV

ROUTINES TO HELP YOU

DEVELOP A DAILY YOGA

PRACTICE

Use the chapters in Part IV to help create your own daily yoga practice. Each chapter provides a series of suggested postures to address a particular issue or complaint: waking up well, relieving tension, recharging your energy, and counteracting stress for better sleep. The postures included here are easy to practice at any time and in (almost) any place. Identify your needs, try the suggested yoga postures, and practice regularly, adding or replacing postures as you gain confidence and an understanding of the most beneficial postures for you.

ENJOY YOGA EVERY DAY

The following exercises are suitable for those beginning a yoga practice. Keep in mind that exercises having beneficial effects also have contraindications. The greatest problem is that beginners often overdo. To perform an exercise in an effective way without harming yourself, you need to be aware of the proper alignment as well as of the proper breathing. The best thing to do: Focus your awareness on the effects of each posture. What does the posture do to your body and your mind? Does it feel good?

Do not forget to include the eye exercises (Chapter 13).

NOTES OF CAUTION

As a reminder, pregnant women should only do yoga exercises tailored to their condition. People with glaucoma, detached retina, ear inflammation, or high blood pressure should keep their head above heart level. If you feel acute pain, do relaxing postures and do not fight the pain. After longer breaks (i.e., injury, sickness, and surgical treatment), slowly restart your yoga practice. If you have an abdominal hernia, any injury, inflammation in your back or abdomen, or sciatica, consult your health care practitioner before you start practicing.

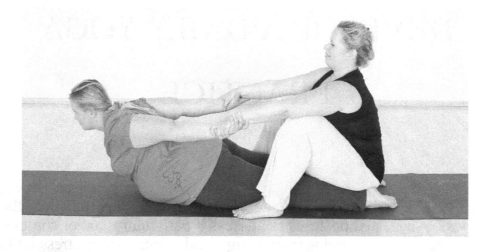

REMEMBER

Inhale and exhale through your nose during the yoga exercises. To develop your own rhythm of practicing yoga, always start the exercises from the same side of the body and repeat the exercises for a constant length. Use a journal that helps you to develop a daily yoga practice. Write down which yoga postures you enjoy most and which postures have a noticeable effect.

HAVE A QUICK LOOK

The following chart helps you to find a suitable yoga posture or set of postures. I also suggest practicing the eye exercises detailed in chapter 13 throughout the day to strengthen your eye muscles and relieve eye strain, itchiness, or blurred vision.

Aims	Set of postures
Chapter 20 To wake up Stretch, ease sore muscles, and prepare for the day	Knees to chest
	Dorsal knee rotation
	Torso rotation
	Palm tree posture
Chapter 21 To realign and relieve tension Relieve joint and muscle tension and improve your mobility	Head rotation
	Arm rotation of bent arms
	Hand lotus
	Hip rotation
	Knee rotation
Chapter 22 To recharge Improve memory and focus and increase your strength and energy	Alternate nostril breathing
	Hero 2 posture
	Hero 1 posture
Chapter 23 To sleep well Relax and prepare for sleep	Legs up the wall
	Crocodile posture
	Yoga nidra

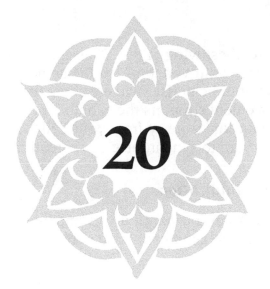

To Wake Up

For a better start to your day, try these gentle stretches first thing in the morning.

KNEES TO CHEST

It is easy to perform knees to chest lying in bed. This exercise gently stretches your spine and widens the spaces between your vertebrae. At the same time, the movement deepens your breath. The pressure in your belly rises while you are moving your knees toward your chest. This phase of the movement supports the exhalation. The pressure in the belly lowers while you are moving your knees away from your belly. This phase of the movement supports the inhalation. It is vital to synchronize your breathing with your movement.

Notes of Caution and Contraindications

This exercise is very gentle. It can be harmful to someone who suffers from abdominal pain. Use a cushion if you want to keep your head above heart level.

Alignments

Keep your neck stretched out and relax your lower legs and feet. Rest your head on a cushion if you suffer from high blood pressure or eye or ear conditions.

What to Do

- Stretch out on your back.
- Bend your knees, and bring them closer to your chest. Place your right hand on your right knee and your left hand on your left knee. Make sure that both your lower legs and feet are relaxed and that your neck is stretched.
- Exhaling through your nose, bend your arms, and pull your knees closer to your chest.

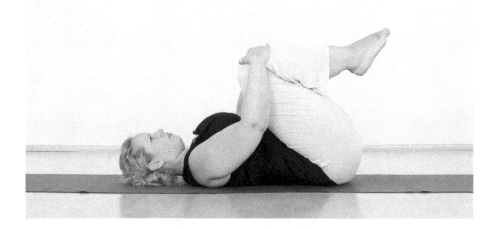

- Inhaling through your nose, stretch your arms, and move your knees away from your chest.

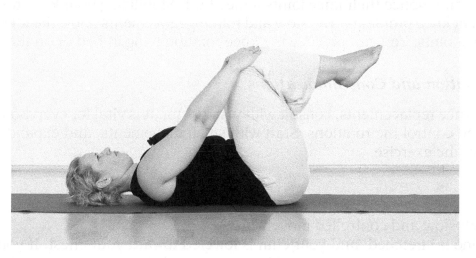

- Repeat the movement during at least six complete inhalations and exhalations.
- Finally, stretch out again, and feel the effects. Close your eyes if you like.

DORSAL KNEE ROTATION

Most people only notice their knee joints if they hurt. Mobilizing your knee rotations helps you to prevent knee problems. The slow and rotating movements allow the alignment of the delicate knee joints. You can practice the knee rotation lying in bed or on the floor.

Notes of Caution and Contraindications

If you have knee replacements, consult with your doctor. It is vital for everybody to exercise with care and control the rotations. Start with small movements, and expand them during the course of the exercise.

Alignments

Exercise with slow and controlled movements.

Your spine is stretched, and your chin is lowered toward your chest. If you suffer from high blood pressure or eye or ear conditions, your head should rest on a cushion or folded blanket.

What to Do

- Stretch out on your back.
- Bend your knees and place your right hand on your right knee and your left hand on your left knee.

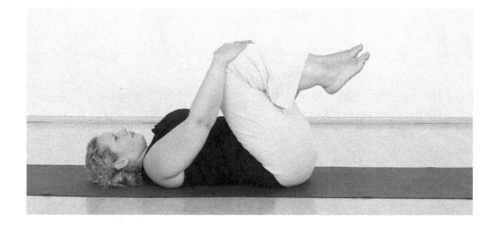

■ Slowly start moving your lower legs in small circles. As you proceed, feel the movements of your knee joints with your palms. Recognize noises and obstructions.

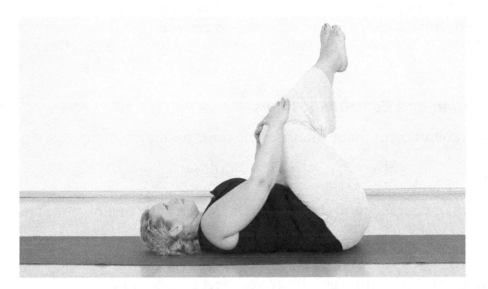

■ Synchronize your breathing with your movement (i.e., inhaling during one rotation, exhaling during one rotation).
■ Repeat the movements during six complete inhalations and exhalations.
■ Continue the exercise rotating in the opposite direction. Notice differences in your knees or differences depending on the direction of the rotation.
■ Finally, lie on your back, and feel the effects of the complete exercise.

TORSO ROTATION

The torso rotation is a very powerful posture, even though it is easy to do and requires little space or time to perform. It aligns and mobilizes many joints, including your spine, shoulders, and arms, making it the perfect posture with which to start your day. If you stand tall with your feet well grounded on your mat, it also mobilizes the joints of your feet, legs, and hip.

Notes of Caution and Contraindications

There are no general contraindications for the torso rotation.

Alignments

The outer sides of your feet and the soles are in fixed contact with your mat.

What to Do

Keep your arms at shoulder height. Place your feet parallel, and make sure that your soles are in full contact with the floor.

- Come into the upright standing posture.
- Place your feet more than hip width apart. Make sure that both soles and both outer sides of your feet are touching the mat.
- Inhaling through your nose, slowly raise both arms and stretch them to your sides at shoulder height. Raise your arms; do not pull up your shoulders. If you are not exactly sure, you can pull up your shoulders briefly and let them sink again.
- Bend your right arm until your hand is in front of your sternum.

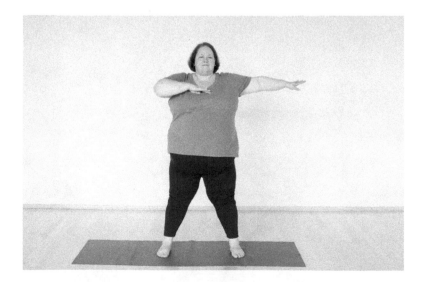

■ Exhaling, turn your outstretched left arm backward and rotate your upper torso and your head to the left, leading with your outstretched left arm.

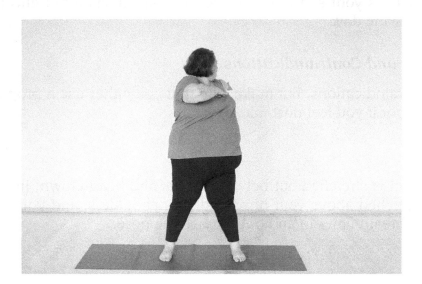

■ Inhaling, rotate back into the starting posture. Change the position of your arms; bend the left arm, and stretch out the right arm.
■ Exhaling, turn your head and upper body to the right, leading with your outstretched right arm.
■ Inhaling, turn back again, changing the positions of your arms, and continue.
■ Repeat this torso rotation six times.
■ With an exhalation, lower your arms.
■ Finally, while in the standing posture, feel the effects of the rotation in your shoulders and upper spine. Close your eyes if it is pleasant for you.

PALM TREE POSTURE

The palm tree posture can provide a first stretch in the morning. It is a gentle but profound stretch that challenges your sense of balance. It is also a small but effective exercise for short breaks during the day.

Notes of Caution and Contraindications

There are no contraindications, but make sure that you either use a prop or practice with both feet on the floor if you feel unstable.

Alignments

Your spinal column is stretched out between pelvis and head crown, including the neck. Your arms are stretched above your head and your shoulders, and your face and tongue are relaxed. Your breath flows in and out through the nose.

What to Do

Your spinal column is stretched out between pelvis and crown, including the neck. Your arms are stretched above your head and shoulders, and your face and tongue are relaxed. Your breath flows in and out through the nose.

- Come into the upright standing posture.
- Cross your fingers, and lay your hands on your head with your palms facing the ceiling.

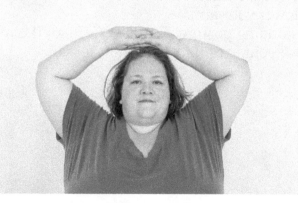

- Inhaling through your nose, stretch your arms and lift your heels until your weight is balanced on the tips of your toes.

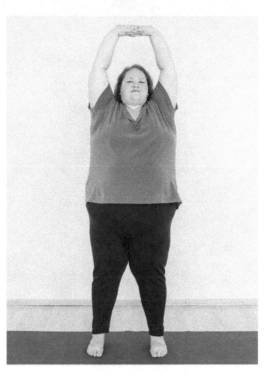

- Exhaling through your nose, lower your arms to your sides, and place your feet back on the mat with the weight evenly spread over your soles.
- Repeat the movement during six complete inhalations and exhalations.
- Finally, return to the standing posture and feel the energy in your feet and the effects of the balancing posture. If it is comfortable, close your eyes.

21

To Relieve Tension

Each of these postures will help mobilize a certain joint or group of joints, easing tension throughout your body.

"Twists and rotations are my favorite yoga exercises. Sometimes my belly gets in the way, but in the end I always find a way to work it out."

—Denise

HEAD ROTATION

The head rotation exercise relieves tension in the neck and shoulders.

Notes of Caution and Contraindications

If you suffer from a painful neck and soreness in your shoulders, start with moderate movements.

Alignments

Keep your chin parallel to the floor while rotating your head. (Do not bow and rotate.)

What to Do

Always start with an inhalation and a stretch of your spine to create space for the vertebrae and discs. On the exhale, do the rotation.

- Sit upright on a chair or on a mat.
- Place your hands on top of your thighs.
- Inhaling, stretch your spinal column and neck.
- Exhaling, relax your shoulders.

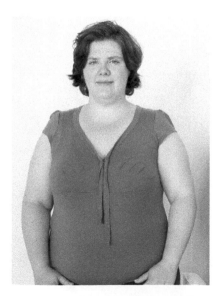

■ Inhaling, turn your head to the left. Make sure that your chin is parallel to the floor and your head does not bow. Keep your shoulders relaxed.

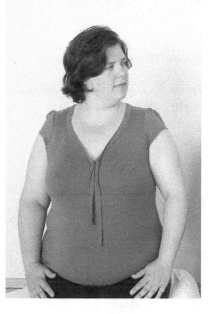

■ Exhaling, turn your head to the right without a bow.

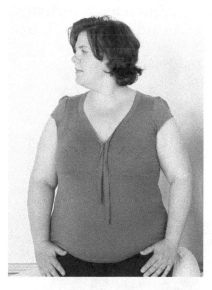

■ Repeat the rotation for six complete inhalations and exhalations.
■ Get back into your initial posture. Feel the effect of the rotations. You may close your eyes if you like.

ARM ROTATION WITH BENT ARMS

Arm rotations counter a tight chest and a round upper back. At the same time, they mobilize the shoulder and arm joints. It is important that you do not hurt yourself by moving too vigorously.

Notes of Caution and Contraindications

It is vital to control the movement if you rotate your extremities. Start with slow, small movements and expand them during the exercise.

Alignments

Keep your shoulders relaxed.

What to Do

Keep your spine in an upright position and your arms fully stretched out at shoulder height.

- Come into the upright seated posture on a chair.
- Place your hands on top of your thighs.
- Inhaling, slowly raise your arms sideways to shoulder height. Make sure that you are raising your arms only, not your shoulders. If you are uncertain, briefly pull up your shoulders and let them sink again.
- Exhaling, bend both arms up so your hands touch the tops of your shoulders.
- Gently rotate your shoulders forward starting with small circles, enlarging them in the course of the exercise.

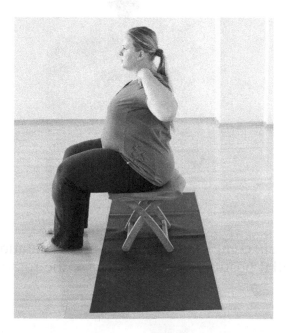

- Keep a steady breathing rhythm that matches the rotations.
- Do the gentle move for at least six inhalations and exhalations in a forward rotation.
- Change the direction, and gently rotate backward for at least six inhalations and exhalations.

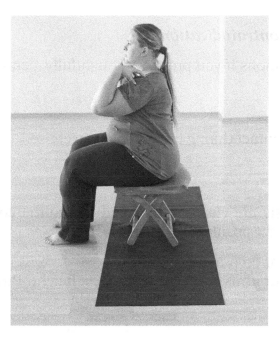

- You can do the exercise with your eyes closed.
- Exhaling, lower your arms. Rest your hands on your thighs, and feel the effects in shoulders and arms.

HAND LOTUS

The lotus exercise is a gentle rotation that bends your wrists and relaxes your fingers. It is a good exercise to counteract soreness in fingers and wrists resulting from long hours of manual work.

Notes of Caution and Contraindications

There are no contraindications if you practice thoughtfully, gently mobilizing the joints.

Alignments

Your wrists are in close contact during the complete exercise.

What to Do

Make sure that your wrists are closely connected during the complete movement. Relax your shoulders in an upright position.

- Sit upright on a chair or on a mat.
- Inhale while lifting your arms and elbows to chest height. Push your palms together.

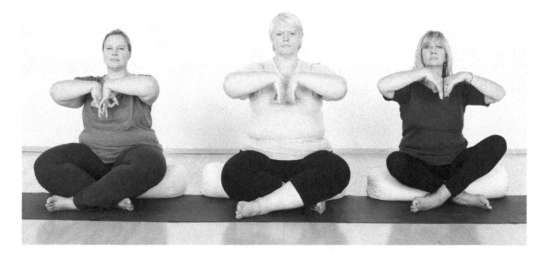

- Put the tips of both your index fingers and thumbs together to form a nice circle and relax the other fingers.
- Gently rotate your hands and forearms outward. Both wrists are moving around one another until the back of your hands meet with your fingers pointing downward.

- Continue the rotation until your fingers point upward again.
- Remain in a breathing rhythm that matches the gentle rotations.
- Continue the gentle movement for six inhalations and exhalations.
- Change the direction, gently rotating your hands and forearms inward for another six inhalations and exhalations.
- You can do the exercise with your eyes closed.
- With an exhalation, lower your arms into your lap, and feel the effects in your wrists.

HIP ROTATION

This exercise mobilizes your hip joints as well as your knees and ankles. Keep both feet firmly on the ground, and slowly extend your movements.

Notes of Caution and Contraindications

There are no contraindications for this exercise.

Alignments

The outer sides of your feet and the soles are in firm contact with your mat.

What to Do

- Come into the upright standing posture.
- Put your feet one leg length apart. Make sure that both soles and both outer sides of your feet are touching the ground. Extend your knees, making sure not to hyperextend them.
- Place your hands on your hips.

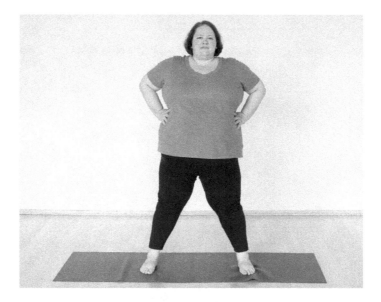

■ Slowly start moving your pelvis in a circle and keep to a steady breathing rhythm. Expand the movement.

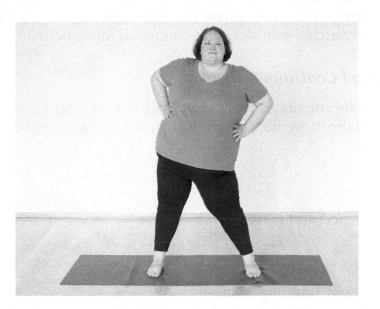

■ After a while, change the direction of the hip rotation and continue the exercise.

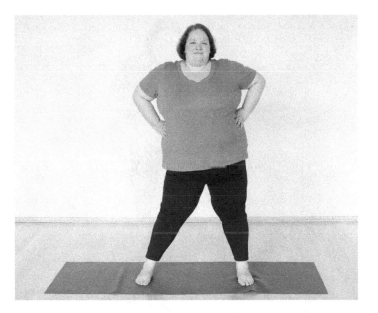

■ Finally, stop the rotation and return to the standing posture. Feel the effects of the steady rotation.

KNEE ROTATION

Knee rotations in a standing posture can be done almost everywhere. By practicing the knee rotations frequently, you will improve the alignment of your knee joints and help prevent knee problems. Exercise with slow and controlled movements.

Notes of Caution and Contraindications

If you have knee replacements, consult your doctor. It is vital for everybody to exercise with care and control the movements. Start with small rotations and expand them over the course of the exercise.

Alignments

Keep your spine stretched and relax your shoulders.

What to Do

- Come into the upright standing posture.
- Bend both your knees and put your hands on top of your kneecaps. Your fingers are facing downward.

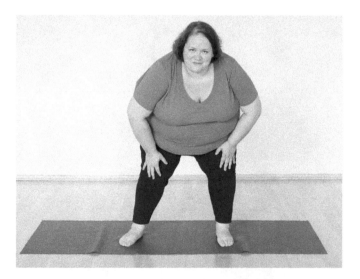

- Fully stretch out your spine, and do not bow your upper torso.
- Slowly rotate your knees in one direction, and keep to a regular breathing rhythm.
- Continue in that direction while you do six complete inhalations and exhalations.
- Change the direction, and do the rotation to the right side during the next six full breath cycles.

■ Gently stop the movement, roll your body upward with your knees bent, and come into the standing posture.

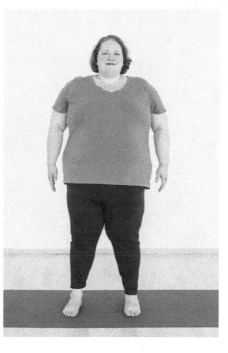

■ Feel the effects in your knees. You may close your eyes if you like.

22

To Recharge

Yoga is a good antidote for sluggishness. These exercises will boost your energy by opening up your airways and improving blood circulation.

ALTERNATE NOSTRIL BREATHING

This small yoga exercise has a wide range of effects: It immediately widens the bronchial tubes, helps you to breathe evenly, relaxes the body, calms the mind, and increases awareness. People suffering from asthma can have very good results.

Notes of Caution and Contraindications

There are no general contraindications for this exercise. Practice with care and consciousness to feel its full benefit. Stop the exercise if you feel dizzy.

Alignments

Sit upright and relax your shoulders. Use a bolster to support your working hand and arm if you like.

What to Do

- Sit on a chair or get into a comfortable posture on your mat.
- Bend the index finger, middle finger, and ring finger of your right hand, and stretch out your thumb and little finger.
- Place your right thumb next to your right nostril and your right little finger next to your left nostril. Either place your bent arm on a table, or hold it comfortably in front of your body so that it is not pushing on your thorax and is not blocking your breathing.
- To begin, first breathe out deeply through both nostrils.
- Close your right nostril with your thumb, and slowly breathe in through your left nostril.

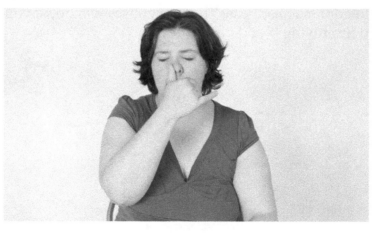

■ Close your left nostril with your little finger, and slowly breathe out completely through your right nostril.

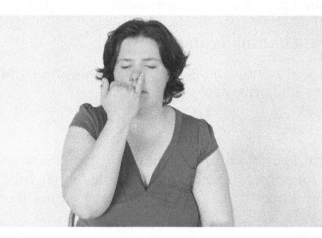

■ Slowly breathe in again through your right nostril. Close your right nostril with your thumb, and slowly breathe out again through your left nostril.
■ Repeat the alternate nostril breathing for at least six complete breath cycles.
■ Finally, lower your hand and breathe in and out through both your nostrils. Feel the calming effects. Keep your eyes closed if you like.

HERO 2 POSTURE

This posture strengthens your foot and leg muscles and improves balance.

Notes of Caution and Contraindications

There are no general contraindications. Be gentle with joints and stay aligned with your knees over your ankles and arms at shoulder height.

Alignments

Stretch your spine and keep your torso centered. Your pelvis and your forward pointing foot are in line. Keep your arms stretched and at shoulder height. The posture is perfect and most beneficial for your knees if your ankles are under your knees.

What to Do

- Come into the upright standing posture.
- Turn your right foot completely outward, and take a step forward in the same direction.
- Turn your left foot 45 degrees inward. Make sure that your pelvis is in the same position it was when you started.
- Inhaling, raise your arms to shoulder height. Stretch out both arms and keep the stretch. Feel the stretch in your arms and in your fingertips.
- Exhaling, slowly bend your right knee forward.
- Turn your head and look over your outstretched right arm. Make sure that your torso is in an upright position; do not bend forward.

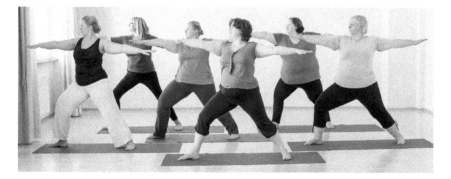

- Keep the position for six full inhalations and exhalations.
- With an inhalation, stretch both legs and lower your arms.
- Bring your feet into the starting position, and compare both sides of your body—both legs, both sides of your pelvis, both shoulders, both sides of your face.
- Repeat the posture with your other foot in front.
- Finally, return to the standing posture, and feel the energy in your body. Close your eyes if you like.

HERO I POSTURE

This posture provides a gentle backbend and works your body from head to toe, strengthening your foot, leg, arm, and shoulder muscles, stretching your whole spine, and mobilizing your shoulder joints.

Notes of Caution and Contraindications

There are no general contraindications for the Hero 1 posture.

Alignments

Keep your feet hip width apart. Align your bent knee with your ankle. Stretch your complete spine, and keep your pelvic muscles tightened.

What to Do

If you practice the hero 1 in motion, breathe and move steadily and rhythmically. Gently bend backward. Completely stretch your spine, leg, and arms, and keep your pelvic muscles tightened.

- Come into the upright standing posture.
- Move your left foot forward. Make sure that your feet are still hip width apart. Keep both legs stretched and both heels on the floor.
- Bring both palms together in front of your sternum.

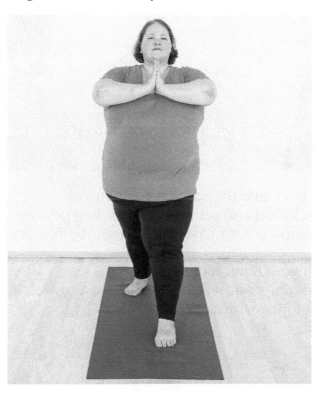

- With an inhalation, slowly bend your front leg while pushing your elbows backward and stretching your shoulders. Make sure that your front knee is properly aligned over your ankle.
- With an exhalation, slowly move back into the starting position with palms together and the front knee stretched.
- Repeat the exercise for six full inhalations and exhalations.
- To keep the posture, inhale, bend your front knee, stretch out your arms and look upward.
- Hold this posture for six full inhalations and exhalations.

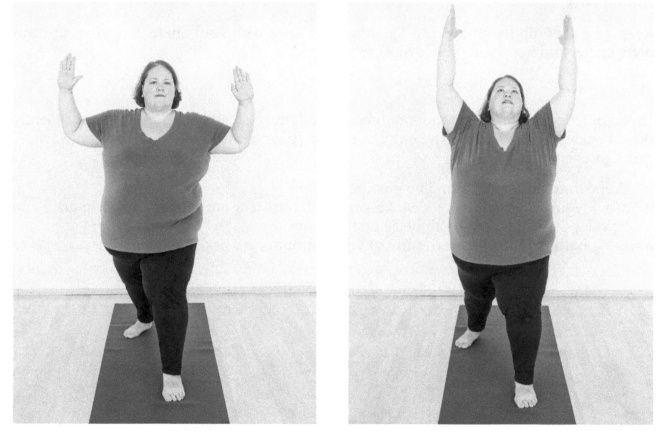

- With an inhalation, get back into the starting position.
- Move your front foot backward and get into the standing posture.
- Close your eyes and compare both sides—both legs, both sides of your pelvis, both sides of your face.
- Repeat the exercise with your other foot in front.
- Finally, return to the standing posture, close your eyes, and feel the stretch of your back and the balancing effect of the whole exercise.

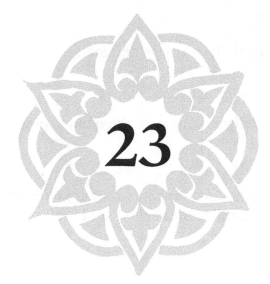

23

To Sleep Well

All the following postures can be practiced while lying in bed. They are a great way to relieve tension before going to sleep. They can also be done any time you feel stressed to help you relax.

LEGS UP THE WALL

This exercise will relieve tension in your legs and feet.

Notes of Caution and Contraindications

Put a cushion under your head if you suffer from high blood pressure or eye or ear conditions.

Alignments

Do not hyperextend your knees. Use blankets to bolster your back and place your head on a cushion if it feels more comfortable and helps you to relax.

What to Do

- Come into a lying posture.
- With an inhalation, slowly move your legs upward against the wall.
- Stretch your spine and place your arms alongside your body.
- Place your heels at the wall.
- Keep the posture for at least six complete inhalations and exhalations.
- With an exhalation, bend your knees and roll to the side.
- Close your eyes if you like.

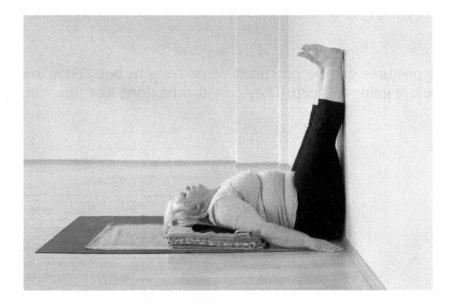

CROCODILE POSTURE

The crocodile posture provides a rotation of the stretched vertebrae and strengthens the belly muscles.

Notes of Caution and Contraindications

The crocodile rotation is contraindicated for pregnant women. Place your head on a cushion if you want to keep your head above heart level.

Alignments

Keep your whole spine stretched and in contact with the mat during the complete movement. Do not forget to stretch your neck and lower your chin toward your chest.

What to Do

- Come into the dorsal starting posture.
- Stretch your entire spine, your legs, and your arms.
- Bend your knees, and place both your feet close together on the ground.
- Place your pelvis further to the left until your weight is on the right side of your bottom. Bend your knees, and lift them toward your chest.
- Exhale while moving the knees completely to the right side and your head to the left side. Make sure that both shoulders are still on the mat and that your neck is stretched.
- Maintain the posture for six complete inhalations and exhalations. You may close your eyes if you like. The more you relax, the easier it is to stay in this posture.
- As you inhale, turn back into the starting position, and compare the feeling in both sides of your body—both legs, both sides of the pelvis, both sides of your shoulders, and both sides of your face.
- Repeat the asana on the other side.
- Finally, stretch out on your back and feel the effect of the complete asana.

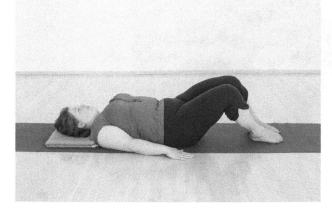

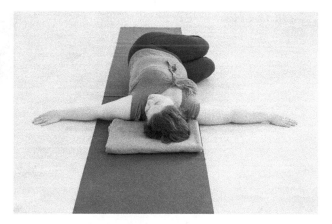

YOGA NIDRA

Yoga nidra is an excellent way to end a set of postures. It can be practiced in bed and function as a very effective preparation for a sound sleep.

Notes of Caution and Contraindications

There are no contraindications for yoga nidra. Place your head on a bolster if you want to keep your head above heart level or if it feels more comfortable.

Alignments

There is no right way of doing yoga nidra; just find a way that works best for you.

What to Do

- Stretch out on your back.
- Rotate your feet to the side.
- Put your arms alongside your body with palms facing the ceiling.
- Relax your shoulders and make sure they are flat on the mat.
- Stretch your neck, and lower your chin toward your sternum.
- Relax your face and mouth muscles.
- Close your eyes. Make sure that you can entirely relax in this position.
- Deeply breathe in and out through your nose.

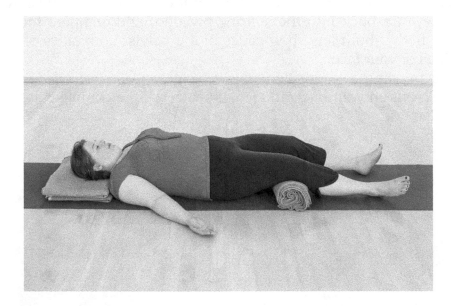

- Bring your attention to your left foot, your left sole, your left ankle, your left lower leg, your left knee, your left thigh, your left hip joint.
- Bring your attention to your right foot, your right sole, your right ankle, your right lower leg, your right knee, your right thigh, your right hip joint.
- Bring your attention to your left hand, your left palm, your left wrist, your left forearm, your left ellbow, your left upper arm, your left shoulder joint.
- Bring your attention to your right hand, your right palm, your right wrist, your right forearm, your right ellbow, your right upper arm, your right shoulder joint.
- Bring your attention to the back of your head where it lies on the mat, to your forehead, to the front of your body, your left brow, your right brow, your left eye, your right eye, the tip of your nose, your upper lip, your lower lip, the tip of your chin.
- Bring your attention to your belly, observing how it moves up and down. Keep your attention on your belly for a couple of inhalations and exhalations. Feel the effects of yoga nidra.

If you want to get up after yoga nidra:

- Completely inhale and exhale through your nose several times.
- Make small movements with your toes and fingers, with your feet and hands, and with your legs and arms. Stretch your body if it feels good.
- Get up into a seated posture, and feel the effects of yoga nidra with your eyes closed.

Resources and Recommended Reading

ON HEALTH, SIZE, AND DIVERSITY

Health at Every Size (HAES®)

www.haescommunity.org

"Health at Every Size is based on the simple premise that the best way to improve health is to honor your body. It supports people adopting health habits for the sake of health and well-being (rather than weight control). Health at Every Size encourages:

- Accepting and respecting the natural diversity of body sizes and shapes.
- Eating in a flexible manner that values pleasure and honors internal cues of hunger, satiety, and appetite.
- Finding the joy in moving one's body and becoming more physically vital."

Association for Size Diversity And Health (ASDAH)

www.sizediversityandhealth.org

"The Association for Size Diversity and Health (ASDAH) is an international professional organization composed of individual members who are committed to the principles of Health at Every Size (HAES). The mission of the Association for Size Diversity and Health (ASDAH) is to promote education, research, and the provision of services which enhance health and well-being, and which are free from weight-based assumptions and weight discrimination."

National Association to Advance Fat Acceptance (NAAFA)

www.naafaonline.com

"Our Goal NAAFA endeavors to ensure that diversity and inclusion is intrinsic to our organization, reflecting the values we wish others to apply to their organizations, businesses and institutions. We also want to unite our members and supporters representing all areas of difference by showing our solidarity of diversity in all its forms. We are committed to adding size diversity to the equation ensuring all people across the size spectrum are valued and respected."

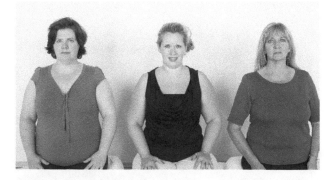

ON YOGA

Below are the websites of ten well-known yoga traditions. I encourage you not to make a decision about what approach is best for you based only on this information. Attend a class and then decide. See Chapter 2 for information on finding the right yoga class.

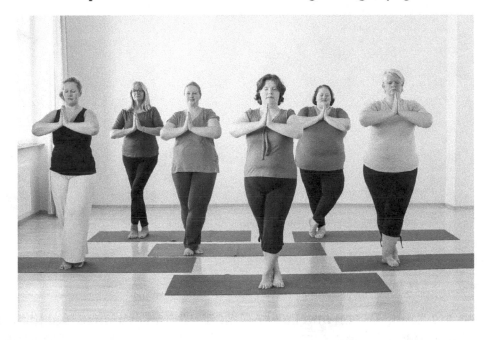

Vini: www.viniyoga.com
Triyoga: www.triyoga.com
Sivananda: www.sivananda.org
Kundalini: www.3ho.org
Jivamukti: www.jivamuktiyoga.com
Iyengar: www.iynaus.org
Gitananda: www.gitanandayogasociety.com
Bikram: www.bikramyoga.com
Ashtanga: www.ashtanga.com
Anusara: www.anusara.com

RECOMMENDED READING

The websites on health, size, and diversity offer long lists of interesting books. Here is a small selection of studies, academic, and popular titles you may also find of interest:

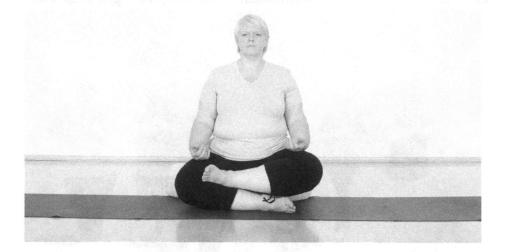

A RECENT STUDY

In a recent study, Linda Bacon and Lucy Aphramor found evidence that the Health at Every Size (HAES)-approach achieves improvements in physiological measures (blood pressure), health behaviors (eating and activity habits), and psychosocial outcomes (self-esteem and body image), more successfully than the dominant weight loss treatment. Read the study here:

Bacon, Linda and Lucy Aphramor. "Weight Science: Evaluating the evidence for a paradigm shift." *Nutrition Journal* 10, no. 9 (2011).

Or online here: http://www.nutritionj.com/content/10/1/9

THEORY BOOKS

Sander L. Gilman is interested in the way societies talk about obesity and the obese. Obesity can be a health problem, disease, personal weakness, moral malice, or social disorder, and a fat man can be a medical case, solid as a rock, or a vulnerable child in a large body, for example. The author presents the diverse cultural meanings attached to obesity and the obese and their connotations: a new worldwide challenge, a national problem, terrifying development, etc.

Gilman, Sander L. *Obesity: The Biography*. New York: Oxford University Press, 2010.

Gilman, Sander L. *Fat: A Cultural History of Obesity*. Cambridge: Polity, 2008.

Gilman, Sander L. (2004): *Fat Boys: A Slim Book*. Lincoln: University of Nebraska Press, 2004.

POPULAR BOOKS

Below are some well-known books by authors who have a positive attitude toward large bodies, encourage people to speak up and question dieting, and are engaged in the work of the anti-discrimination movement.

Erdman, Cheri. *Live Large! Affirmations for Living the Life You Want in the Body You Already Have.* Carlsbad: Gurze Books, 2003.

Frater, Lara. *Fat Chicks Rule!: How to Survive in a Thin-Centric World.* Gamble Guides, 2005.

Gaesser, Glenn. *Big Fat Lies: The Truth about Your Weight and Your Health.* New York: Fawcett, 1996.

Hillman, Carolyn. *Love Your Looks: How to Stop Criticizing and Start Appreciating Your Appearance.* New York: Touchstone, 1996.

Johnson, Carol A. *Self-Esteem Comes in All Sizes.* Carlsbad: Gurze Books, 1996.

Newman, Leslea. *SomeBody to Love: A Guide to Loving the Body You Have.* Chicago: Third Side Press, 1991.

Shanker, Wendy. *The Fat Girl's Guide to Life.* New York: Bloomsbury, 2005.

Wann, Marilyn. *Fat! So? Because You Don't Have to Apologize for Your Size.* New York: Ten Speed Press, 1998.

Notes

1. p. 4: *Studies have found that the ruling focus on weight loss is ineffective* … Linda Bacon and Lucy Aphramor, "Weight Science: Evaluating the Evidence for a Paradigm Shift," *Nutrition Journal 10, no. 9* (January 24, 2011).

2. p. 8: *You should pay particular attention to* … Carrie Peyton Dahlberg, "Living Large," *Yoga Journal* (December 2000): 90. An encouraging article for students and teachers of size.

3. p. 9: *Appropriate responses to a class* … Mara Carrico, *Yoga Basics: The Essential Beginner's Guide to Yoga for a Lifetime of Health and Fitness* (New York: Henry Holt, 2007): 38–39. This is a solid companion for beginners who want to learn the essentials of a posture. It only gives very few modified versions of the detailed postures.

4. p. 11: *Once you are able to achieve a certain posture* … Dietrich Ebert, "Western Medicine and Yoga," *The Yoga Path, 4th ed.* (Petersberg Germany: Via Nova, 2003): 275–285. *The Yoga Path* is a manual written by more than 30 members of the German yoga association.

5. p. 172: *Being Awake and Being Asleep chart.* Ingrid Kollak, In *Yoga for Nurses*, by Ingrid Kollak. (New York: Demos Health, 2009): 189. This book addresses typical work-life situations, well-known health problems, and including yoga in your self-care.

Index